ICD-10-CM CODING CONCEPTS

A Review Guide - 2023 Version

Lisa L. Campbell, Ph.D.

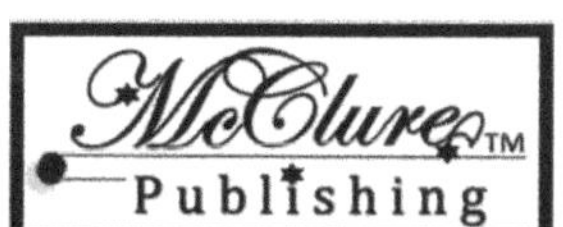

McClure Publishing, Inc.
www.McClurePublishing.com

To order additional copies, please contact:

McClure Publishing, Inc.
www.mcclurepublishing.com
800.659.4908

Lisa L. Campbell, Ph.D.
Physician Practice Resources, Inc.
www.drlisalcampbell.org
855.737.5472

ICD-10-CM Coding Concepts: A Review Guide

2023 Version

Dr. Lisa L. Campbell, PhD

Table of Contents

Chapter 1-Introduction, Conventions & General Guidelines 1

Introduction to the ICD-10-CM Guidelines 1
Conventions for the ICD-10-CM 3
General Coding Guidelines 9
Chapter 2-Chapter Specific Guidelines 20

Certain Infectious and Parasitic Disease (A00-B99, U07.1) 20
Neoplasms (C00-D49) 32
Endocrine, Nutritional and Metabolic Diseases (E00-E89) 39
Mental and Behavioral Disorders (F01-F99) 42
Diseases of Nervous System and Sense Organs (G00-G99) 45
Diseases of the Eye and Adnexa (H00-H59) 48
Diseases of the Circulatory System (I00-I99) 50
Diseases of Respiratory System (J00-J99, U07.0) 58
Diseases of Skin and Subcutaneous Tissue (L00-L99) 61
Diseases of Musculoskeletal System and Connective Tissue (M00-M99) 64
Diseases of Genitourinary System (N00-N99) 66
Pregnancy, Childbirth, and the Puerperium (O00-O9A) 67
Newborn (Perinatal) Guidelines (P00-P96) 77
Congenital Malformations, Deformations/Chromosomal Abnormalities (Q00-Q99) 82
Symptoms, Signs and Abnormal Clinic and Laboratory Findings, NEC (R00-R99) 84
Injury, Poisoning and Certain Other Consequences of External Causes (S00-T88) 87
External Causes of Morbidity (V01-Y99) 98
Factors Influencing Health Status and Contact with Health Service (Z00-Z99) 105
Chapter 3-Selection of Principal and Secondary Diagnosis 115

Chapter 4-Outpatient Coding Guidelines 121

Answer Key 128

Chapter 1-Conventions and General Coding Guidelines 129
Chapter 2-Chapter Specific Coding Guidelines 134
Chapter 3-Selection of Principal and Secondary Diagnoses 163
Chapter 4-Outpatient Coding and Reporting 165

About the Author

Dr. Campbell is a multi-faceted health care professional with 30 years of experience. Having a passion for working with physician practices, Dr. Campbell enjoys helping providers improve their operational effectiveness with a focus on documentation integrity.

She holds professional memberships with the American Health Information Management Association (AHIMA), American Academy of Professional Coders (AAPC), American College of Healthcare Executives (ACHE) and the Healthcare Compliance Association (HCCA).

She holds a Masters in Health Administration (MHA), Masters in Project Management (MPM) and Doctor of Philosophy (PhD) degree in Health Care Administration. Additionally, she holds the following nationally recognized credentials:

- Registered Health Information Administrator (RHIA)
- Certified Documentation Improvement Practitioner (CDIP)
- Certified Coding Specialist (CCS)
- Certified Coding Specialist-Physician Based (CCS-P)
- Certified in Healthcare Compliance (CHC)
- Certified Professional Coder (CPC)
- Certified Outpatient Coder (COC)
- Certified Professional Biller (CPB)
- Certified Risk Coder (CRC)
- Certified Professional Medical Auditor (CPMA)
- Certified Professional Coder-Instructor (CPC-I)

Lastly, Dr. Campbell has been an educator since 1997 on-campus and online, for several Colleges and Universities across the United States.

Chapter 1-Introduction, Conventions & General Guidelines

Introduction to the ICD-10-CM Guidelines

1. The ICD-10-CM is a morbidity classification published by the United States for classifying diagnoses and reason for visits in all health care settings.

    a.   True
    b.   False

2. List the four organizations that make up the cooperating parties for the ICD-10-CM system:

    a.   ____

    b.   ____

    c.   ____

    d.   ____

3. The instructions and conventions of the classification do not take precedence over the guidelines.

    a.   True
    b.   False

4. These guidelines are based on the _____________ and ________________ instructions in the tabular list and alphabetic index but provide additional instruction.

5. Adherence to the ICD-10-CM guidelines is required under _____________________.

6. A joint effort between the healthcare _____________ and _____________ is essential to achieve complete and accurate documentation, code assignment, and reporting of diagnoses and procedures.

7. The entire _______________ should be reviewed to determine the specific reason for the encounter and the conditions treated.

8. The term encounter is used for all settings, including _____________________________.

9. The term provider is used throughout the guidelines to mean physician or any qualified health care practitioner who is legally accountable for establishing the patient's ____.

10. The official guidelines are organized into (4) sections, which can be identified:

 a. Section I

  1. ____

  2. ____

  3. ____

 b. Section II____

 c. Section III____

 d. Section IV____

11. It is not necessary to review all sections of the guidelines to fully understand all of the rules and instructions needed to code properly.

 a. True
 b. False

Conventions for the ICD-10-CM

12. The conventions, general guidelines and chapter-specific guidelines are applicable to _______ healthcare settings unless otherwise indicated.

13. The conventions for the ICD-10-CM are the general rules for use of the classification __________________ of the guidelines.

14. The ICD-10-CM is divided into the_____________________ ___________________, an alphabetical list of terms and their corresponding code, and the ____________ __________________ a structured list of codes divided into chapters based on body system or condition.

15. The Alphabetic Index consists of the following parts:

     a. ____

     b. ____

     c. ____

     d. ____

16. The ICD-10-CM Tabular List contains categories, subcategories and codes.

     a. True
     b. False

17. Codes may be _______, _______, _______, _______ or _______ characters.

18. A code that has an applicable 7th character is considered __________ without the 7th character.

19. What type of format does ICD-10-CM use for ease in reference? ______________

20. For reporting purposes only codes are permissible, not __________________ or ______________________________, and any applicable 7th character is required.

21. The ICD-10-CM utilizes a placeholder character _______, which is used as a placeholder at certain codes to allow for future expansion.

22. Where a placeholder exists, the X must be used in order for the code to be considered a valid code.

    a.   True
    b.   False

23. The 7th character must always be the _________ character in the data field.

24. If a code that requires a 7th character is not 6 characters, a placeholder ______ must be used to fill in the empty characters.

25. What does the abbreviation "Not elsewhere classifiable" (NEC) represent when found in the Alphabetic Index?

    ____

26. What does the abbreviation "Not otherwise specified" (NOS) represent when found in the Alphabetic Index?

    ____

27. What does the abbreviation "Not elsewhere classifiable" (NEC) represent when found in the Tabular List?

    ____

28. What does the abbreviation "Not otherwise specified" (NOS) represent when found in the Tabular List?

    ____

29.   Explain the purpose of the following punctuation.

  a.   Brackets ____

  ____

  b.   Parentheses____

  ____

  ____

  ____

  c.   Colon ____

  ____

30.   Codes titled "other" or "other specified" are for use when the information in the medical record provides detail for which a specific ______________ does not exist.

31.   Codes titled "unspecified" are for use when the information in the medical record is insufficient to assign a more ______________ code.

32.   The ______________ ______________ appears immediately under a three character code title to further define, or give examples of, the content of the category.

33.   Inclusion terms are list of terms included under some codes, these terms are the conditions for which that code is to be used, but are not necessarily exhaustive.

  a.   True
  b.   False

34.   The ICD-10-CM has ______________ types of excludes notes, each type of note has a ______________ definition for use but they are all similar in that they indicate that codes excluded from each other are independent of each other.

35.   A type 1 Excludes note is a pure exclusion note, it means not coded here. An Excludes 1 note indicates ____

____

36.   An Excludes 1 is used when __________ conditions cannot occur together.

37.   An exception to the Excludes 1 definition is the circumstance when the two conditions are ______________to each other.

38.   A type 2 Excludes note represents, not included here, it indicates that the condition ________________ is not part of the condition represented by the code, but a patient may have __________ conditions at the same time.

39.   When an Excludes2 note appears under a code, it is _________________ to use both the code and the excluded code together, when appropriate.

40.   Certain conditions have both an underlying etiology and multiple body system manifestations due to the underlying etiology. For such conditions, the ICD-10-CM has a coding convention that requires the underlying condition be sequenced first, if applicable, followed by the _______________________________________.

41.   As it relates to the previous question, whenever such a combination code exists, there is a "________________________________" note at the etiology code, and a "code first" note at the ___________________ code.

42.   "In diseases classified elsewhere" codes are never permitted to be used as first-listed or ___________________ diagnosis.

43.   In the Alphabetic Index when both conditions are listed together, the etiology code is reported first followed by the manifestation codes in brackets, the code in brackets is always to be sequenced second.

   a.   True
   b.   False

44.   The word "and" should be interpreted to mean either "___________________" or "___________________", when it appears in a title.

45. The word "with" or "in" should be interpreted to mean "associated with" or "______________________" when it appears in a code title, the Alphabetical index (either under a main term or subterm), or an instructional note in the Tabular list.

46. The classification does not presume a causal relationship between the two conditions linked by the terms "associated with" or "due to" in the Alphabetic Index or Tabular List.

    a. True
    b. False

47. As it relates to the previous question, these conditions should be coded as related even in the absence of provider documentation explicitly linking them, unless the documentation clearly states the conditions are unrelated or when another guideline exists that specifically requires a documented linkage between two conditions.

    a. True
    b. False

48. For conditions not specifically linked by these relational terms in the classification or when a guideline requires that a linkage between two conditions be explicitly documented, provider documentation must link the conditions in order to code them as related.

    a. True
    b. False

49. The word "with" in the Alphabetical Index is sequenced immediately following the main term, not in alphabetical order.

    a. True
    b. False

50. The "see" instruction following a main term in the Alphabetic index indicates that another term should be ______________________.

51.   As it relates to the previous question, it is necessary to go to the main term referenced with the "see" note to locate the correct code.

    a.   True
    b.   False

52.   A "see also" instruction following a main term in the Alphabetical Index instructs that there is another main term that may also be referenced that may provide additional Alphabetic Index ______________ that may be useful.

53.   It is not necessary to follow the "see also" note when the original main term provides the necessary code.

    a.   True
    b.   False

54.   The ________ __________note instructs that two codes may be required to fully describe a condition, but this note does not provide sequencing direction. The sequencing depends on the circumstances of the __________________.

55.   A code that is listed next to a main term in the ICD-10-CM alphabetical index is referred to as a _______________________   _______________________________

56.   The default code represents that condition that is most commonly associated with the ________________ term, or is the __________________ code for the condition.

57.   If a condition is documented in a medical record without any additional information, ________________________   _______________________________

58.   The assignment of a diagnosis code is based on the provider's diagnostic ________________ that the condition exists.

59.   The provider's statement that the patient _____ a particular condition is sufficient.

60.   Code assignment is not based on clinical criteria used by the provider to establish the diagnosis.

    a.   True
    b.   False

General Coding Guidelines

61. To select a code in the classification that corresponds to a diagnosis or reason for the visit documented in a medical record, first locate the term in the

_______________________________ _____________________ and then verify the code

in the _______________________ ________________________.

62. _________________ and be _____________ by instructional notations that appear in both the Alphabetic Index and the Tabular List.

63. It is essential to use both the Alphabetic Index and the Tabular List when locating and assigning _______________.

64. The alphabetic Index does not always provide the full code, selection of the full code, including laterality and any applicable 7th character can only be done in the

_____________________ _______________________.

65. A dash (-) at the end of an Alphabetical Index entry indicates that additional characters are _______________________.

66. Even if a dash is not included at the Alphabetical Index entry, it is necessary to refer to the _____________ _____________ to verify that no 7th character is required.

67. _______________codes are to be used and reported at their highest number of characters available.

68. A three-character code is to be used only if it is not further subdivided.

    a. True
    b. False

69. A code is invalid if it has not been coded to the full number of characters required for that code, including the 7th character, if applicable.

    a. True
    b. False

70. The appropriate code or codes from ____ must be used to identify diagnoses, symptoms, conditions, problems, complaints or other reason(s) for the encounter/visit.

71. Signs and symptoms, as opposed to a diagnosis are acceptable for reporting purposes when a related definitive ____________________ has not be described (confirmed) by the provider.

72. Chapter __________ of ICD-10-CM, Symptoms, Signs, and Abnormal Clinical and Laboratory Findings, Not Elsewhere Classified (codes R00.0 - R99) contains many, but not all, codes for symptoms.

73. Signs and symptoms that are associated routinely with a disease process should not be assigned as an additional code, unless otherwise instructed by the classification.

    a.   True
    b.   False

74. Additional signs and symptoms that may not be associated routinely with a disease process should be coded when present.

    a.   True
    b.   False

75. "Use additional code" notes are found in the Tabular List at codes that are not part of an etiology/manifestation pair where a secondary code is useful to fully describe a condition.

    a.   True
    b.   False

76. A "use additional code" note will normally be found at the ____________________ disease code, indicating a need for the organism code to be added as a secondary code.

77. When there is a code first note and an underlying condition is present, the underlying condition should be reported second, if known.

    a.   True
    b.   False

78. Code, if applicable, any causal condition first notes indicate that this code may be assigned as a principal diagnosis when the _________________ condition is unknown or not applicable.

79. Multiple codes may be needed for _________________, _________________ codes and _________________ codes to more fully describe a condition.

80. If the same condition is described as both acute (subacute) and chronic, and separate subentries exist in the Alphabetical Index at the same indention level, code _______________ and sequence the _______________ _____________ code first.

81. A combination code is a single code used to classify:

    a.   ____

    b.   ____

    c.   ____

82. Combination codes are identified by referring to sub-term entries in the alphabetic index ____

    ____

83. Assign only the combination code when that code fully identifies the diagnostic conditions _____________ or when the Alphabetic Index directs so.

84. Multiple coding should not be used when the classification provides a combination code that clearly identifies all of the elements documented in the diagnosis.

    a.   True
    b.   False

85. When the combination code lacks necessary specificity in describing the manifestations or complication, an additional code should be used as a secondary code.

    a.   True
    b.   False

86.   A ___________________ is the residual effect after the acute phase of an illness or injury has terminated.

87.   There is a time limit on when a sequela code can be used.

    a.   True
    b.   False

88.   Coding of a sequela generally requires two codes which are sequenced how?

    a.   ____

    ____

    b.   ____

    ____

89.   An exception to the sequela guidelines are for those instances where the code for the sequela is followed by ____

    ____

    ____

90.   The code for the acute phase of an illness or injury that led to the sequela is never used with a code for the sequela.

    a.   True
    b.   False

91. Code any condition described at the time of discharge as "impending" or "threatened" as follows:

    a. If it did occur, code as ____

    b. If it did not occur, reference the alphabetical Index to determine if the condition has a subentry term for "impending" or "threatened" and also reference main term entries for "___________" and for "______________"

    c. If the sub-terms are listed, assign the given ________________.

    d. If the sub-terms are not listed, code the existing underlying condition (s) and not the condition described as ______________ or ________________.

92. Each unique ICD-10-CM diagnosis code can only be reported once per encounter.

    a. True
    b. False

93. Some ICD-10-CM codes indicate laterality, specifying whether the condition occurs on the ____________ ____________ or is ___________________.

94. If no bilateral code is provided and the condition is bilateral, assign separate codes for both the left and right side.

    a. True
    b. False

95. If the side is not identified in the medical record, assign the code for the ______________ side.

96. When a patient has a bilateral condition and each side is treated during separate encounters, assign the "_________________" code, including the encounter to treat the first side.

97. For the second encounter for treatment after one side has previously been treated and the condition no longer exists on that side, assign the appropriate _________________ code for the side where the condition still exists.

98. The bilateral code would not be assigned for the subsequent encounter, as the patient no longer has the condition in the previously treated side.

    a.   True
    b.   False

99. If the treatment on the first side did not completely resolve the condition, then the bilateral code would still be appropriate.

    a.   True
    b.   False

100. Code assignment is based on documentation by patient's provider.

    a.   True
    b.   False

101. As it relates to the previous question, there are a few exceptions, for the Body Mass Index (BMI), depth of non-pressure chronic ulcers, pressure ulcer stage, coma scale, and NIH stroke scale (NIHSS), Social determinants of health (SDOH), laterality, blood alcohol level and underimmunization status, code assignment may be based on medical record documentation from clinicians who are not the patient's provider.

    a.   True
    b.   False

102. Based on the previous question, the associated diagnosis must be documented by the patient's provider.

    a.   True
    b.   False

103. If there is conflicting medical record documentation, either from the same clinician or different clinicians, the patient's attending provider should be queried for clarification.

    a.   True
    b.   False

104. For social determinants of health, code assignment may be based on medical record documentation from _________________ involved in the care of the patient who are not the patient's _________________ since this information represents social information, rather than a medical diagnosis.

105. If there is conflicting medical record documentation, either from the same clinician or different clinicians, the patient's attending provider should be queried for clarification.

    a.   True
    b.   False

106. BMI, coma scale, NIHSS, blood alcohol level, codes for social determinants of health and underimmunization status should only be reported as principal or first-listed diagnoses codes.

    a.   True
    b.   False

107. Follow the _____________________ index guidance when coding syndromes; in absence of the Alphabetic index guidance, assign codes for the documented manifestations of the syndrome.

108. As it relates to the previous question, additional codes for manifestations that are not an _____________________ part of the disease process may also be assigned when the condition does not have a unique code.

109. Code assignment for complications of care is based on the provider's documentation of the _______________________________ between the condition and the care or procedure, unless otherwise instructed by the classification.

110. It is important to note that all conditions that occur during or following medical care or surgery are classified as complications.

    a.   True
    b.   False

111. There must be a cause-and-effect relationship between the care provided and the condition documentation must support that the condition is clinically significant.

   a.   True
   b.   False

112. It is necessary for the provider to explicitly document the term complication.

   a.   True
   b.   False

113. If the provider documents a "borderline" diagnosis at the time of discharge, the diagnosis is coded as confirmed, unless the classification provides a specific entry.

   a.   True
   b.   False

114. Since borderline conditions are not ___________________ diagnoses, no distinction is made between the care setting.

115. Sign/symptom and "unspecified" codes have ___________________, even necessary, uses.

116. If a definitive diagnosis has not been established by the end of the encounter, it is appropriate to report codes for sign(s) and/or symptom(s) in lieu of a definitive diagnosis.

   a.   True
   b.   False

117. When sufficient clinical information isn't known or available about a particular health condition to assign a more specific code, it is acceptable to report the appropriate "___________________" code.

118. Unspecified codes should be reported when they are the codes that most accurately reflect what is known about the patient's condition at the time of that particular encounter.

   a.   True
   b.   False

119. It would be appropriate to select a specific code that is not supported by the medical record documentation or conduct medically unnecessary diagnostic testing in order to determine a more specific code.

    a. True
    b. False

120. An _________________ cause of morbidity code should be assigned to identify the cause of the injury (ies) incurred as a result of the hurricane.

121. The use of external cause of morbidity codes is _______________ to the application of ICD-10-CM codes.

122. External cause of morbidity codes are _______________ to be recorded as a principal diagnosis, the appropriate injury code should be sequenced before any external cause codes.

123. The external cause of morbidity codes capture:

    a. ____

    b. ____

    c. ____

    d. ____

    e. ____

124. External cause codes should be assigned for encounters to treat hurricane victims' medical conditions when no injury, adverse effect or poisoning is involved.

    a. True
    b. False

125. External cause of morbidity codes should be assigned for each encounter for care and treatment of the injury.

    a. True
    b. False

126. External cause of morbidity codes may be assigned in all health care settings.

    a.   True
    b.   False

127. For the purpose of capturing complete and accurate ICD-10-CM data in the aftermath of the hurricane, a healthcare setting should be considered as any location where medical care is provided by licensed healthcare professionals.

    a.   True
    b.   False

128. Codes for _____________________________ events, such as a hurricane, take priority over all other external cause codes except child and adult abuse and terrorism and should be sequenced before other external cause of injury codes.

129. Assign as _________________ external cause of morbidity codes as necessary to fully explain each cause.

130. For injuries incurred as a direct result of the _______________, assign the appropriate code(s) for the injuries, followed by the code X37.0-, Hurricane (with the appropriate 7th character), and any other applicable external cause of injury codes.

131. Code X37.0- also should be assigned when an injury is incurred as a result of flooding caused by a _________________ breaking related to the hurricane.

132. Code X38.-, Flood (with the appropriate 7th character), should be assigned when an injury is from _________________ resulting directly from the storm.

133. Code X36.0.-, Collapse of dam or man-made structure, should not be assigned when the cause of the collapse is due to the hurricane.

    a.   True
    b.   False

134. Use of code X36.0- is limited to collapses of man-made structures due to earth surface movements, not due to storm surges directly from a hurricane.

    a.   True
    b.   False

135. For injuries that are not a direct result of the hurricane, such as an evacuee that has incurred an Injury as a result of a motor vehicle accident, assign the appropriate external cause of morbidity code(s) to describe the cause of the injury, but do not assign code X37.0-, Hurricane.

    a.   True
    b.   False

136. If it is not clear whether the injury was a direct result of the _____________ assume the injury is due to the hurricane and assign code X37.0-, Hurricane, as well as any other applicable external cause of morbidity codes.

137. Z codes may be assigned as appropriate to further _____________ the reasons for presenting for healthcare services, including transfers between healthcare facilities.

Chapter 2-Chapter Specific Guidelines

Certain Infectious and Parasitic Disease (A00-B99, U07.1)

Human Immunodeficiency Virus (HIV) Infections

1.   How would the following condition be coded "Possible HIV infection"?

____

2.   Confirmation does require documentation of positive serology or culture for HIV.

    a.   True
    b.   False

3.   If a patient has a HIV-related condition, what would be the principal and secondary diagnosis?

    a.   ____

    b.   ____

4.   If the reason for admission is hemolytic-uremic syndrome associated with HIV syndrome associated with HIV disease, the principal diagnosis is code _________.

5.   If a patient has a condition unrelated to the HIV-related disease, what would be the principal and secondary diagnosis?

    a.   ____

    b.   ____

6.   The date the patient was diagnosed with HIV is relevant to the sequencing decision.

    a.   True
    b.   False

7. Z21 (Asymptomatic Human Immunodeficiency Virus) infection status, is to be applied when the patient without any documentation of symptoms is listed as being:

    a. ____

    b. ____

    c. ____

    d. ____

8. As it relates to the previous question, do not use Z21, if the term "AIDS" is used or if the patient is treated for any HIV-related illness or is described as having any condition(s) resulting from his/her HIV positive status; use B20 in these cases.

    a. True
    b. False

9. Under which circumstances would you use code R75?

    ____

    ____

    ____

10. Patients with any known prior diagnosis of a HIV-related illness should be coded to ____

11. Once a patient has developed a HIV-related illness, the patient should always be assigned code B20 on every subsequent admission/encounter.

    a. True
    b. False

12. Patient's previously diagnosed with any HIV illness (B20) should never be assigned to R75 or Z21.

  a.   True
  b.   False

13. During pregnancy, childbirth or the puerperium, if a patient is admitted (or presenting for a healthcare encounter) because of a HIV-related condition, what is the principal and secondary diagnosis?

  a.   ____

  b.   ____

14. Which codes are used if an asymptomatic patient is admitted during pregnancy, childbirth or the puerperium for HIV?

  a.   ____

  b.   ____

15. If a patient is being seen to determine his/her HIV status, which code should be used?

  ____

16. If a patient with _______________or _____________ is being seen for HIV testing, code the signs and symptoms.

17. What code is used when a patient returns to be informed of his/her HIV test results? ____

18. If a patient with documented HIV disease, HIV-related illness or AIDS is currently managed on antiretroviral medications, assign code B20, Human immunodeficiency virus [HIV] disease.

  a.   True
  b.   False

19. Certain infections are classified in chapters other than Chapter 1 and no organism is identified as part of the infection code. In these instances, it is not necessary to use an additional code from Chapter 1 to identify the organism.

   a. True
   b. False

20. Many bacterial infections are resistant to current antibiotics, it is not necessary to identify all infections documented as antibiotic resistant.

   a. True
   b. False

21. For a diagnosis of sepsis assign the appropriate code for the underlying systemic inflection, if the type of infection or casual organism is not further specified, assign code ____________.

22. A code from subcategory R65.2, Severe sepsis, should not be assigned unless severe ____________ or an associated acute ________________ dysfunction is documented.

23. Negative or inconclusive blood cultures do not preclude a diagnosis of sepsis in patients with clinical evidence of the condition; however, the provider should be queried.

   a. True
   b. False

24. The term urosepsis is a ________________________________, it is not to be considered synonymous with sepsis.

25. If a patient has sepsis and associated acute organ dysfunction or multiple organ dysfunction (MOD), coders should follow the instructions for coding __________ ____________________.

26. If a patient has sepsis and an acute organ dysfunction, but the medical record documentation indicates that the acute organ dysfunction is related to a medical condition other than the sepsis, assign a code from subcategory R65.2, Severe sepsis.

   a. True
   b. False

27. An acute organ dysfunction must be associated with sepsis in order to assign the ____.

28. The coding of severe sepsis requires a minimum of 2 codes.

   a. True
   b. False

29. If the causal organism is not documented, assign code A41.9, Sepsis, unspecified, for the infection.

   a. True
   b. False

30. Due to the complex nature of severe sepsis, some cases may require querying the provider prior to assignment of these codes.

   a. True
   b. False

31. Septic shock generally refers to circulatory failure associated with severe sepsis, and therefore, it ____

   ____

32. For cases of septic shock, which codes should be sequenced first and second?

   a. ____

   b. ____

33. The code for septic shock, can be assigned as a principal diagnosis.

    a.   True
    b.   False

34. If severe sepsis is present on admission, and meets the definition of principal diagnosis, the underlying systemic infection code should be assigned as the principal diagnosis, followed by ____

____

35. A code from subcategory R65.2 can never be assigned as a principal diagnosis.

    a.   True
    b.   False

36. When severe sepsis develops during the encounter (it was not present on admission), the underlying systemic infection and appropriate code from subcategory _________________should be assigned as_____________________

37. Severe sepsis may be present on admission but the diagnosis may not be _________________ until sometime after admission.

38. If the reason for admission is both sepsis or severe sepsis and a localized infection, what are the principal and secondary diagnoses?

    a.   ____

    b.   ____

39. If the patient is admitted with a localized infection, and sepsis/severe sepsis doesn't develop until after admission, what are the principal and secondary diagnoses?

    a.   ____

    b.   ____

40. As with all postprocedural complications, code assignment is based on the provider's documentation of the relationship between the ________________ and the ____________________.

41. For infections following a procedure, a code from T81.40 to T81.43, or a code from O86.00 to O86.03, that identifies the site of the infection should be coded first, if known, followed by an additional code for sepsis, as well as a code for the infectious agent.

   a.   True
   b.   False

42. If the patient has severe sepsis, the appropriate code from subcategory R65.2 should also be assigned with the additional code(s) for any acute organ dysfunction.

   a.   True
   b.   False

43. For infections following infusion, transfusion, therapeutic injection, or immunization, a code from subcategory T80.2, Infections following infusion, transfusion, and therapeutic injection, or code T88.0-, Infection following immunization, should be coded first, followed by the code for the specific ____________________.

44. If a postprocedural infection has resulted in postprocedural septic shock, assign the codes indicated above for sepsis due to a postprocedural infection, followed by code T81.12-, Postprocedural septic shock. Do not assign code R65.21, Severe sepsis with septic shock.

   a.   True
   b.   False

45.	If sepsis or severe sepsis is documented as associated with a non-infectious condition and this condition meets the definition for principal diagnosis, what is sequenced first and second?

	a.	____

	b.	____

46.	If the infection meets the definition of principal diagnosis, it should be sequenced before the ____

47.	When both the associated non-infectious condition and the infection meet the definition of principal diagnosis, either may be assigned as principal diagnosis.

	a.	True
	b.	False

48.	Only one code from Category R65 should be assigned, therefore, when a non-infectious condition leads to an infection resulting in severe sepsis, do not additionally assign____

49.	If the reason for admission is hemolytic-uremic syndrome that is associated with sepsis, assign code D59.31, Infection-associated hemolytic-uremic syndrome, as the principal diagnosis.

	a.	True
	b.	False

50.	When a patient is diagnosed with an infection that is due to methicillin resistant *Staphylococcus aureus* (MRSA), and that infection has a combination code that includes the causal organism assign the appropriate combination ____________.

51.	When there is documentation of a current infection due to MRSA, and that infection does not have a combination code that includes the causal organism, assign the appropriate code to identify the condition along with code __________

52.	The condition or state of being colonized or carrying MSSA or MRSA is called, ________________________________ or ________________________________ while an individual person is described as being colonized or being a carrier.

53.   Colonization means that MSSA or MRRA is present on or in the body without necessarily causing illness.

   a.   True
   b.   False

54.   A positive MRSA colonization test might be documented by the provider as "MRSA screen positive" or "MRSA nasal swab positive".

   a.   True
   b.   False

55.   Assign code ______________________________ for patients documented as having MRSA colonization.

56.   Assign code ______________________________ for patients documented as having MSSA colonization.

57.   Colonization is not necessarily indicative of a disease process or as the cause of a specific condition the patient may have unless documented as such by the provider.

   a.   True
   b.   False

58.   If a patient is documented as having both MRSA colonization and infection during a hospital admission, code Z22.322, Carrier or suspected carrier of Methicillin resistant Staphylococcus aureus, and a code for the MRSA infection may both be assigned.

   a.   True
   b.   False

59.   Code only a __________________ diagnosis of Zika virus (A92.5, Zika virus disease) as documented by the provider.

60. In this context, "confirmation" does not require documentation of the type of test performed; the physician's diagnostic statement that the condition is confirmed is sufficient.

a. True
b. False

61. If the provider documents "suspected", "possible" or "probable" Zika, do not assign code A92.5. Assign a code(s) explaining the reason for encounter (such as fever, rash, or joint pain) or Z20.821, Contact with and (suspected) exposure to Zika virus.

a. True
b. False

62. Code only a _________________ diagnosis of the 2019 novel coronavirus disease (COVID-19) as documented by the provider or documentation of a positive COVID-19 test result.

63. For a confirmed diagnosis, assign code U07.1, COVID-19.

a. True
b. False

64. In this context, "confirmation" does not require documentation of a positive test result for COVID-19; the provider's documentation that the individual has COVID-19 is sufficient.

a. True
b. False

65. If the provider documents "suspected," "possible," "probable," or "inconclusive" COVID-19, do not assign code U07.1, instead, code the signs and symptoms reported.

a. True
b. False

66. When COVID-19 meets the definition of principal diagnosis, code ___________ should be sequenced first, followed by the appropriate codes for associated manifestations, except when another guideline requires that certain codes be sequenced first, such as obstetrics, sepsis, or transplant complications.

67. When the reason for the encounter/admission is a respiratory manifestation of COVID-19, assign code U07.1, as the principal/first-listed diagnosis and assign code(s) for the respiratory manifestation(s) as ___________________diagnoses.

68. For a patient with acute bronchitis confirmed as due to COVID-19, assign codes ______________ and _____________.

69. Bronchitis not otherwise specified due to COVID-19 should be coded using code _____________ and _______________.

70. If the COVID-19 is documented as being associated with a lower respiratory infection, not otherwise specified (NOS), or an acute respiratory infection, NOS, codes ___________ and ___________________.

71. If the COVID-19 is documented as being associated with a respiratory infection, NOS, codes _________________ and _________________.

72. For acute respiratory distress syndrome (ARDS) due to COVID-19, assign codes _________________ and _________________.

73. For acute respiratory failure due to COVID-19, assign code _________________ and _______________.

74. When the reason for the encounter/admission is a non-respiratory manifestation of COVID-19, assign code U07.1, COVID-19, as the principal/first-listed diagnosis and assign code(s) for the manifestation(s) as additional diagnoses.

    a. True
    b. False

75. For _________________ individuals with actual or suspected exposure to COVID-19, assign code Z20.828, Contact with and (suspected) exposure to other viral communicable diseases.

76. For _________________ individuals with actual or suspected exposure to COVID-19 and the infection has been ruled out, or test results are inconclusive or unknown, assign code Z20.828, Contact with and (suspected) exposure to other viral communicable diseases.

77. For patients presenting with any signs/symptoms associated with COVID-19 but a definitive diagnosis has not been established, assign the appropriate code(s) for _____________ of the presenting signs and symptoms.

78. If a patient with signs/symptoms associated with COVID-19 also has an actual or suspected contact with or exposure to COVID-19, assign Z20.828, Contact with and (suspected) exposure to other viral communicable diseases, as an additional code.

    a.   True
    b.   False

79. For patients with a history of COVID-19, assign code Z86.19, Personal history of other infectious and parasitic diseases.

    a.   True
    b.   False

80. For individuals who previously had COVID-19 and are being seen for follow-up evaluation, and COVID-19 test results are negative, assign codes _____________ and _______________.

81. For an encounter for antibody testing that is not being performed to confirm a current COVID-19 infection, nor is a follow-up test after resolution of COVID-19, assign _________________.

Neoplasms (C00-D49)

1. To properly code a neoplasm it is necessary to determine from the record if the neoplasm is:

    a. ____

    b. ____

    c. ____

    d. ____

2. A primary malignant neoplasm that overlaps two or more contiguous (next to each other) sites should be classified to the subcategory/code .8 ('overlapping lesion'), unless ____

    ____

3. For multiple neoplasms of the same site that are not contiguous, codes for each site should be assigned.

    a. True
    b. False

4. Malignant neoplasms of _________________________________ are to be coded to the site mentioned.

5. The neoplasm table in the Alphabetical Index should be consulted first if the histological term is documented.

    a. True
    b. False

6. The _______________________________should be referenced to verify that the correct code has been selected from the table and that a more specific site code does not exist.

7. If the malignancy is chiefly responsible for occasioning the patient admission/encounter and treatment is directed at the primary site, designate the primary _____________________ as the principal/first-listed diagnosis.

8. The only exception to the guideline in the previous question is if a patient admission/encounter is solely for the administration of chemotherapy, immunotherapy or radiation therapy, assign the appropriate _________ code as the first-listed or principal diagnosis, and the diagnosis or problem for which the service is being performed as a secondary diagnosis.

9. If the patient is admitted for a primary neoplasm with metastasis and treatment is directed toward the secondary site only, what is the principal or first listed diagnosis? ____

____

10. When admission/encounter is for management of anemia associated with the malignancy, and the treatment is only for anemia, which code would be sequenced first and which would be sequenced second?

    First-listed____

    Secondary____

11. When admission/encounter is for management of an anemia associated with an adverse effect of the administration of chemotherapy or immunotherapy and the only treatment is for the anemia, how would this situation be sequenced?

    First-listed____

    Secondary____

    Tertiary____

12. When the admission/encounter is for management of anemia associated with an adverse effect of radiotherapy, the anemia code should be sequenced first, followed by the appropriate neoplasm code and code _______________________________

13. When admission/encounter is for management of dehydration due to the malignancy and only dehydration is being treated (intravenous rehydration), which code would be sequenced first and which would be sequenced second?

    First-listed____

    Secondary____

14. When admission/encounter is for treatment of a complication resulting from a surgical procedure performed, what is the principal or first listed diagnosis?

    ____

15. When a primary malignancy has been previously excised or eradicated from its site and there is no further treatment directed to that site and there is no evidence of any existing primary malignancy at that site, a code from category Z85, Personal history of malignant neoplasm, should be used to indicate the former site of the malignancy.

    a. True
    b. False

16. Any mention of extension, invasion, or metastasis to another site is coded as a _________________________________ malignant neoplasm to that site.

17. When an episode of care involves the surgical removal of a neoplasm, primary or secondary site, followed by adjunct chemotherapy or radiation treatment during the same episode of care, the code for the _______________________ should be assigned as principal or first-listed diagnosis.

18. If a patient admission/encounter is solely for the administration of chemotherapy, immunotherapy or external beam radiation therapy, the following codes be assigned:

    Radiation therapy____

    Chemotherapy____

    Immunotherapy____

19.   If a patient admission/encounter is for the insertion or implantation of radioactive elements (e.g., brachytherapy) the appropriate code for the malignancy is sequenced as the principal or first-listed diagnosis; code Z51.0 should not be assigned.

   a.   True
   b.   False

20.   When the patient is admitted for the purpose of external beam radiotherapy, immunotherapy or chemotherapy and develops complications such as uncontrolled nausea and vomiting or dehydration, what should be coded as principal or first-listed?

   a.   ____

   b.   ____

   c.   ____

21.   When a patient is admitted for the purpose of insertion or implantation of radioactive elements (e.g., brachytherapy) and develops complications such as uncontrolled nausea and vomiting or dehydration, the principal or first-listed diagnosis is the appropriate code for the ______________________________ followed by any codes for the complications.

22.   When the reason for admission/encounter is to determine the extent of the malignancy, or for a procedure such as paracentesis or thoracentesis, the primary malignancy or appropriate ___________________ site is designated as the principal or first-listed diagnosis, even though chemotherapy or radiotherapy is administered.

23.   Symptoms, signs, and ill-defined conditions listed in Chapter 18 characteristic of, or associated with, an existing primary or secondary site malignancy can be used to replace the malignancy as principal or first-listed diagnosis.

   a.   True
   b.   False

24. A patient cannot have more than one malignant tumor in the same organ.

    a. True
    b. False

25. Code C80.0 is for use only in those cases where the patient has an advanced metastatic disease and no known primary or secondary sites are specified.

    a. True
    b. False

26. C80.1 equates to cancer unspecified.

    a. True
    b. False

27. If the reason for the encounter is for treatment of a primary malignancy, coders should assign the _______________________ as the principal or first-listed diagnosis.

28. When an encounter is for a primary malignancy with metastasis and treatment is directed toward the metastatic site, which site is designated as principal or first-listed? ____

29. When a pregnant woman has a malignant neoplasm, a code from subcategory O9A.1- should be sequenced first, followed by the appropriate code from Chapter 2 to indicate the type of neoplasm.

    a. True
    b. False

30. When an encounter is for management of a complication associated with a neoplasm and the treatment is only for the complication, the complication is coded second.

    a. True
    b. False

31. When the admission/encounter is for management of an anemia associated with the malignancy, and the treatment is only for anemia, the appropriate code for the malignancy is sequenced as the principal or first-listed diagnosis followed by code ________________________________.

32. When an encounter is for treatment of a complication resulting from a surgical procedure performed for treatment of the neoplasm, designate the complication as the ____

33. When an encounter is for a pathological fracture due a neoplasm and the focus of the treatment is the fracture, a code from subcategory ___________________ should be sequenced first, followed by ______________________________

34. If the focus of treatment is the neoplasm with an associated pathological fracture, the ___________________ should be sequenced first, followed by a code for the ____

35. When a primary malignancy has been excised but further treatment is directed toward that site, then the primary malignancy code should be used until treatment is completed.

    a. True
    b. False

36. When a primary malignancy has been previously excised or eradicated from its site, there is no further treatment directed to that site, and there is no evidence of any existing malignancy at that site, which category code is used? ____________________

37. Subcategories Z85.0 – Z85.85 should only be assigned for the former site of a primary malignancy, not the site of a ___________malignancy.

38. Codes from subcategory Z85.89, may be assigned for the former site(s) of either a _________________ or _____________ malignancy included in this subcategory.

39. When coding leukemia and multiple myeloma, the provider should be queried if the documentation is unclear as to whether or not the patient is in remission.

    a. True
    b. False

40.   A malignant neoplasm of a ______________________ organ should be coded as a transplant complication, assign first the appropriate code from category ________, Complications of transplanted organs and tissue, followed by code ______________________ Malignant neoplasm associated with transplanted organ. Lastly, use an additional code for the specific ________________.

41.   When a malignant neoplasm of lymphoid tissue metastasizes beyond the lymph nodes, a code from categories C81-C85 with a final character ______________ should be assigned identifying "extranodal and solid organ sites" rather than a code for the secondary neoplasm of the affected solid organ.

Endocrine, Nutritional and Metabolic Diseases (E00-E89)

Diabetes Mellitus

1. The diabetes mellitus codes are combination codes that include the:

    a. ____

    b. ____

    c. ____

2. Diabetes codes should be sequenced based on the _________________ for a particular encounter.

3. Assign as many codes from categories E08-E13 as needed to identify all of the associated conditions that the patient has.

    a. True
    b. False

4. The age of the patient is the sole determining factor in determining the type of diabetes.

    a. True
    b. False

5. When the type of diabetes mellitus is not documented in the medical record, the default type is? ____

6. If the patient is treated with both oral hypoglycemic drugs and insulin, both code Z79.4, Long term (current) use of insulin, and code Z79.84, Long term (current) use of oral hypoglycemic drugs, should be assigned.

    a. True
    b. False

7. If the patient is treated with both oral hypoglycemic drugs and insulin, only the code for long-term (current) use of ________________ should be assigned.

8. If the patient is treated with both insulin and an injectable non-insulin antidiabetic drug, assign codes ________________ and ________________.

9. If the patient is treated with both oral hypoglycemic drugs and an injectable non-insulin antidiabetic drug, assign codes ________________ and ________________.

10. Code Z79.4 should not be assigned if insulin is given temporarily to bring a type 2 patient's blood sugar under control during an encounter.

    a. True
    b. False

11. An underdose of insulin due to an insulin pump failure should be assigned which two codes:

    a. ____

    b. ____

12. An overdose of insulin due to an insulin pump failure should be assigned the following two codes:

    a. ____

    b. ____

13. Codes under Category E08, E09 and E13, identify complications or manifestations associated with ________________ diabetes mellitus.

14. Secondary diabetes is not caused by another condition or event.

    a. True
    b. False

15. For patients with secondary diabetes mellitus who routinely use insulin or oral hypoglycemic drugs, an additional code from category _______________should be assigned to identify the long-term (current) use of insulin or oral hypoglycemic drugs.

16. If the patient is treated with _________________ oral medications and insulin, only the code for long-term (current) use of insulin should be assigned.

17. The sequencing of the secondary diabetes codes in relationship to codes for the cause of the diabetes is based on ____

____

18. For postpancreatectomy diabetes mellitus, which three codes should be assigned?

    a. ____

    b. ____

    c. ____

19. Secondary diabetes may be caused by an adverse effect of correctly administered medications, poisoning or sequela of poisoning.

    a. True
    b. False

Mental and Behavioral Disorders (F01-F99)

1.   Assign code F45.41, for pain that is exclusively related to psychological disorders.

    a.   True
    b.   False

2.   Code F45.42, Pain disorders with related psychological factors, should be used with a code from ____

3.   Selection of codes describing "in remission" for categories F10-F19, Mental and behavioral disorders due to psychoactive substance use requires the provider's
____

4.   Mild substance use disorders in early or sustained remission are classified to the appropriate codes for substance abuse in ____________________________, and moderate or severe substance use disorders in early or sustained remission are classified to the appropriate codes for substance dependence in remission.

5.   When the provider's documentation refers to use, abuse and dependence of the same substance (e.g. alcohol, opioid, cannabis, etc.), only one code should be assigned to identify the pattern of use based on the following hierarchy:

    a.   ____

   ____

    b.   ____

   ____

    c.   ____

   ____

    d.   ____

   ____

6. As with all other unspecified diagnoses, the codes for unspecified psychoactive substance use (F10.9-, F11.9-, F12.9-, F13.9-, F14.9-, F15.9-, F16.9-, F18.9-, and F19.9-) should only be assigned based on provider documentation and when they meet the definition of a reportable diagnosis.

    a. True
    b. False

7. Medical conditions due to substance use, abuse, and dependence are not classified as substance-induced disorders

    a. True
    b. False

8. A code from category Y90, Evidence of alcohol involvement determined by blood alcohol level, may be assigned when this information is documented and the patient's provider has documented a condition classifiable to category F10, Alcohol related disorders.

    a. True
    b. False

9. The blood alcohol level does need to be documented by the patient's provider for it to be coded.

    a. True
    b. False

10. For patients with documented factitious disorder on self or Munchausen's syndrome, assign the appropriate code from subcategory F68.1-, Factitious disorder imposed on self.

    a. True
    b. False

11.   Munchausen's syndrome by proxy (MSBP) is a disorder in which a caregiver (perpetrator) falsely reports or causes an illness or injury in another person (victim) under his or her care, such as a child, an elderly adult, or a person who has a disability.

    a.   True
    b.   False

12.   As it relates to the previous condition, this condition is also referred to as "factitious disorder imposed on another" or "factitious disorder by proxy." The perpetrator, not the victim, receives this diagnosis.

    a.   True
    b.   False

13.   Assign code ______________, Factitious disorder imposed on another, to the perpetrator's record.

14.   For the victim of a patient suffering from MSBP, assign the appropriate code from categories ____________, Adult and child abuse, neglect and other maltreatment, confirmed, or ____________, Adult and child abuse, neglect and other maltreatment, suspected.

15.   The ICD-10-CM classifies dementia (categories F01, F02, and F03) based on the etiology and severity, which is defined as, ________________________________,

________________, ______________________________ and __________________.

16.   If the documentation does not provide information about the severity of the dementia, assign the appropriate code for ____________________ severity.

17.   If a patient is admitted to an inpatient acute care hospital or other inpatient facility setting with dementia at one severity level and it progresses to a higher severity level, assign one code for the lowest severity level reported during the stay.

    a.   True
    b.   False

Diseases of Nervous System and Sense Organs (G00-G99)

1. Codes from category G81, Hemiplegia and hemiparesis, and subcategories, G83.1, Monoplegia of lower limb, G83.2, Monoplegia of upper limb, and G83.3, Monoplegia, unspecified, identify _______________________________________

    ____

2. Should the affected side be documented, but not specified as dominant or nondominant, and the classification system does not indicate a default, code selection is as follows:

    a. ____

    ____

    b. ____

    ____

    c. ____

    ____

3. Codes in Category G89, Pain, not elsewhere classified, may be used in conjunction with codes from other categories and chapters to provide more detail about:

    a. ____

    b. ____

4. If the pain is not specified as acute or chronic, post-thoracotomy, postprocedural or neoplasm-related, do not assign codes from category ________________.

5. A code from category G89 should not be assigned if the underlying diagnosis is known, unless the reason for the encounter is pain control/management and not management of the ____.

6. When an admission or encounter is for a procedure aimed at treating the underlying condition, a code for the underlying condition should be assigned as the _________________________________ diagnosis.

7. Category G89 codes are acceptable as principal diagnosis or the first-listed code when:

    a. ____

    ____

    ____

    b. ____

    ____

    ____

    ____

8. Codes from Category G89 may be used in conjunction with codes that identify the site of pain if category G89 provides additional __________________.

9. The sequencing of category G89 codes with site-specific pain codes (including chapter 18 codes), is dependent on the circumstances of the encounter/admission, if the encounter is for pain control or pain management, assign which two codes:

    a. ____

    b. ____

10. If the encounter is for any other reason except pain control or pain management, and a related definitive diagnosis has not been established (confirmed) by the provider, assign the code for the specific site of the pain first, followed by ____.

11. The _________________ documentation should be used to guide the coding of postoperative pain.

12. For post-thoracotomy pain and other postoperative pain not specified as acute or chronic, code for the ____.

13. Routine or expected postoperative pain immediately after surgery should be coded.

    a. True
    b. False

14. Postoperative pain not associated with a specific postoperative complication is assigned to the appropriate ____

15. Postoperative pain associated with a specific postoperative complication is assigned to ____

16. Chronic pain is classified to subcategory ____

17. Code _________________ is assigned to pain documented as being, associated or due to cancer, primary or secondary malignancy, or tumor.

18. G89.3 may be assigned as the principal or first-listed code when the stated reason for the admission/encounter is documented as pain _________________/____.

19. When the reason for the admission/encounter is management of the neoplasm and the pain associated with the neoplasm is also documented, G89.3 may be assigned as an additional diagnosis.

    a. True
    b. False

20. Central pain syndrome (G89.0) and chronic pain syndrome (G89.4) are different than the term "chronic pain," and therefore this code should only be used when the provider has specifically documented this condition.

    a. True
    b. False

Diseases of the Eye and Adnexa (H00-H59)

1. Assign as many codes from category H40, Glaucoma, as needed to identify the

    a. ____

    b. ____

    c. ____

2. When a patient has bilateral glaucoma and both eyes are documented as being the same type and stage, and there is a code for bilateral glaucoma, report only

    ____

    ____

3. When a patient has bilateral glaucoma and both eyes are documented as being the same type and stage, and the classification does not provide a code for bilateral glaucoma report only ____

    ____

    ____

4. When a patient has bilateral glaucoma and each eye is documented as having a different type or stage, and the classification distinguishes laterality, assign the appropriate code for each eye rather than the code for bilateral glaucoma.

    a. True
    b. False

5. When a patient has bilateral glaucoma and each eye is documented as having a different type, and the classification does not distinguish laterality, assign one code for each type of glaucoma with the appropriate the ______ character for the stage.

6.   When a patient has bilateral glaucoma and each eye is documented as having the same type, but different stage, and the classification does not distinguish laterality, assign a code for the type of glaucoma for each eye with the seventh character for the specific glaucoma stage documented for each eye.

   a.   True
   b.   False

7.   If a patient is admitted with glaucoma and the stage progresses during the admission, assign the code for lowest stage documented.

   a.   True
   b.   False

8.   Assignment of the seventh character "4" for "indeterminate stage" should be based on the ____.

9.   Based on the previous question, the seventh character "4" is used for glaucoma's whose stage cannot be _________________ determined.

10.   Based on the previous two questions, this seventh character should not be confused with the seventh character _____ which should be assigned when there is no documentation regarding the stage of the glaucoma.

11.   If "blindness" or "low vision" of both eyes is documented but the visual impairment category is not documented, assign code H54.3, Unqualified visual loss, both eyes.
   a.   True
   b.   False

12.   If "blindness" or "low vision" in one eye is documented but the visual impairment category is not documented, assign a code from H54.6-, unqualified visual loss, one eye.

   a.   True
   b.   False

13.   If "blindness" or "visual loss" is documented without any information about whether one or both eyes are affected, assign code H54.7, Unspecified visual loss.

   a.   True
   b.   False

Diseases of the Circulatory System (I00-I99)

1.   ICD-10-CM classification system presumes a causal relationship between hypertension and heart involvement and between hypertension and kidney involvement, as the two conditions are linked by the term "with" in the Alphabetic Index.

   a.   True
   b.   False

2.   As it relates to question 1, these conditions should be coded as related even in the absence of provider documentation explicitly linking them, unless the documentation clearly states the conditions are unrelated.

   a.   True
   b.   False

3.   For hypertension and conditions not specifically linked by relational terms such as "with," "associated with" or "due to" in the classification, provider documentation must link the conditions in order to code them as related.

   a.   True
   b.   False

4.   __________________ with heart conditions classified to I50. - or I51.4-I51.7, I51.89, I51.9, are assigned to a code from category I11, Hypertensive heart disease.

5.   Patients assigned to a code within Category I11, Hypertensive heart disease, should also be assigned a code from category _________, to identify the type of heart failure in those patients with heart failure.

6.   The same heart conditions (I50. - or I51.4-I51.7, I51.89, I51.9) with hypertension are coded separately if the provider has specifically documented a different cause; sequence according to the circumstances of the admission/encounter.

   a.   True
   b.   False

7.   Assign codes from category I12, Hypertensive chronic kidney disease, when both hypertension and a condition classifiable to category N18, Chronic kidney disease (CKD) are _____________________.

8.   _____________ should not be coded as hypertensive if the physician has specifically documented a different cause.

9.   The appropriate code from category _________ should be used as a secondary code with a code from category I12 to identify the stage of chronic kidney disease.

10.   If a patient has ____ and acute renal failure, an additional code for the acute renal failure is required.

11.   Assign codes from combination category I13, Hypertensive heart and chronic kidney disease, where there is _________________ with both __________ and _________ involvement.

12.   The appropriate code from category N18, Chronic kidney disease, should be used as a secondary code with a code from category I13 to identify the stage of chronic kidney disease.

      a.   True
      b.   False

13.   The codes in category I13, Hypertensive heart and chronic kidney disease, are _____________________ codes that include hypertension, heart disease and chronic kidney disease.

14.   The Includes note at I13 specifies that the conditions included at I11 and I12 are included together in I13. If a patient has hypertension, heart disease and chronic kidney disease, then a code from ____________ should be used, not individual codes for hypertension, heart disease and chronic kidney disease, or codes from I11 or I12.

15.   For patients with both acute renal failure and chronic kidney disease, the acute renal failure should also be _______________, sequence according to the circumstances of the admission/encounter.

16. When the diagnosis of hypertensive cerebrovascular disease is documented, what two codes are required?

    First-listed____

    Second____

17. Subcategory H35.0, Background retinopathy and retinal vascular changes, should be used with a code from category I10 – I15, Hypertensive disease to include the systemic hypertension; the ___________________ is based on the reason for the encounter.

18. When the diagnosis of secondary hypertension is documented, what two codes are assigned?

    a. ____

    b. ____

19. Assign code R03.0, elevated blood pressure reading without a diagnosis of hypertension, unless patient has an established diagnosis of ______________.

20. Assign code O13.-, Gestational [pregnancy-induced] hypertension without significant proteinuria, or O14.-, Pre-eclampsia, for transient hypertension of pregnancy.

    a. True
    b. False

21. Hypertension, controlled usually refers to an existing state of hypertension under ______________ by therapy; assign the appropriate code from categories I10-I15, Hypertensive diseases.

22. Uncontrolled hypertension may refer to untreated hypertension or hypertension not ___________________ to current therapeutic regimen; in either case, assign the appropriate code from categories I10-I15, Hypertensive diseases.

23. Assign a code from category I16, Hypertensive crisis, for documented hypertensive____________, hypertensive ___________or unspecified hypertensive crisis. Code also any identified hypertensive disease (I10-I15); the sequencing is based on the ______________ for the encounter.

24. Pulmonary hypertension is classified to category I27, Other pulmonary heart diseases. For secondary pulmonary hypertension (I27.1, I27.2-), code also any associated conditions or adverse effects of drugs or toxins, the ______________ is based on the reason for the encounter, except for adverse effects of drugs.

25. ICD-10-CM uses combination codes for atherosclerotic heart disease with angina pectoris; which includes subcategories:

   a. ____

   b. ____

26. As it relates to the previous question, when using one of these combination codes (I25.11 and I25.7) it is not necessary to use an additional code for angina pectoris.

   a. True
   b. False

27. A causal relationship can be assumed in a patient with both ________________ and angina ________________, unless the documentation indicates the angina is due to something other than the atherosclerosis.

28. If a patient with ______________________________ is admitted due to an acute myocardial infarction (AMI), the AMI should be sequenced before the coronary artery disease.

29. Medical record documentation does not need to clearly specify the cause-and-effect relationship between the medical intervention and the cerebrovascular accident in order to assign a code for intraoperative or postprocedural cerebrovascular accident.

   a. True
   b. False

30. As it relates to the previous question, proper code assignment depends on whether it was an infarction or hemorrhage and whether it occurred intraoperatively or postoperatively, if it was a cerebral hemorrhage, code assignment depends on the ________________ of procedure performed.

31. Category I69, Sequelae of cerebrovascular is used to indicate complications classifiable to categories ______-______ as the causes of sequela themselves classified elsewhere.

32. As it relates to the previous question, these "late effects" include neurologic deficits that persist after initial ____________ of conditions classifiable to categories I60-I67.

33. The neurologic deficits caused by cerebrovascular disease may be present from the ____________ or may _________ at any time after the onset of the condition classifiable to categories I60-I67.

34. Codes from category I69, Sequelae of cerebrovascular disease, that specify hemiplegia, hemiparesis, and monoplegia identify whether the _______________ or ____________________ side is affected.

35. Should the affected side be documented, but not specified as dominant or nondominant, and the classification system does not indicate a default, code selection is as follows:

    a. ____

    b. ____

    c. ____

36. Codes from category I69 may be assigned on a health record with codes from I60-I67, if the patient has a current cerebrovascular disease and ______________ from an old cerebrovascular disease.

37. Codes from category I69 should not be assigned if the patient does not have neurologic deficits.

    a. True
    b. False

38. The ICD-10-CM codes for type 1 acute myocardial infarction (AMI) identify the site.

    a. True
    b. False

39.   Subcategories I21.0-I21.2 and code ___________ are used for ST elevation myocardial infraction (STEMI).

40.   Code _________is used for non-ST elevation myocardial infarction (NSTEMI) and nontransmural MIs.

41.   If a type 1 NSTEMI evolves to STEMI, assign the_______________________ code.

42.   If type 1 STEMI converts to NSTEMI due to thrombolytic therapy, it is still coded as STEMI.

   a.   True
   b.   False

43.   For encounters occurring while the myocardial infarction is equal to, or less than, four weeks old, including transfers to another acute setting or a post-acute setting, and the myocardial infarction meets the definition of "other diagnoses", codes from category I21 may continue to be reported.

   a.   True
   b.   False

44.   For encounters after the 4 weeks (28 days) time frame and the patient requires continued care related to the myocardial infarction, the appropriate aftercare code should be assigned, rather than a code from category I21.

   a.   True
   b.   False

45.   For old or healed myocardial infarctions not requiring further care, code _________________ may be assigned.

46.   Code I21.9, Acute myocardial infarction, unspecified, is the default for unspecified acute myocardial infarction or unspecified type.

   a.   True
   b.   False

47. If only _________________ STEMI or transmural MI without the site is documented, assign code I21.3, ST elevation (STEMI) myocardial infarction of unspecified site.

48. If an AMI is documented as nontransmural or subendocardial, but the site is provided, it is still coded as a ____

49. A code from category I22, Subsequent ST elevation (STEMI) and non-ST elevation (NSTEMI) myocardial infarction, is to be used when a patient who has suffered a type 1 or unspecified AMI has a new AMI within the __________ week time frame of the initial AMI.

50. A code from category I22 must be used in conjunction with a code from category I21.

    a. True
    b. False

51. The sequencing of the I22 and I21 codes does not change based on circumstances of the encounter.

    a. True
    b. False

52. Do not assign code _____________________________ for subsequent myocardial infarctions other than type 1 or unspecified.

53. For subsequent type 2 AMI assign only code _________________.

54. For subsequent type 4 or type 5 AMI, assign only code _________________.

55. If a subsequent myocardial infarction of one type occurs within 4 weeks of a myocardial infarction of a different type, assign the appropriate codes from category _______ to identify each type, do not assign a code from I22.

56. Codes from category __________ should only be assigned if both the initial and subsequent myocardial infarctions are type 1 or unspecified.

57. Type _______ myocardial infarctions are assigned to codes I21.0-I21.4 and I21.9.

58.   Type _______myocardial infarction (myocardial infarction due to demand ischemia or secondary to ischemic balance) is assigned to code I21.A1, Myocardial infarction type 2 with a code for the underlying cause.

59.   Do not assign code I24.8, Other forms of acute ischemic heart disease, for the ________________ ischemia.

60.   Sequencing of type 2 AMI or the underlying cause is dependent on the ___________________ of admission.

61.   When a type 2 AMI code is described as NSTEMI or STEMI, only assign code ________________.

62.   Codes I21.01-I21.4 should only be assigned for type 1 AMIs.

   a.   True
   b.   False

63.   Acute myocardial infarctions type 3, 4a, 4b, 4c and 5 are assigned to code I21.A9, Other myocardial infarction type.

   a.   True
   b.   False

64.   The "Code also" and "Code first" notes should not be followed related to complications, and for coding of postprocedural myocardial infarctions during or following cardiac surgery.

   a.   True
   b.   False

Diseases of Respiratory System (J00-J99, U07.0)

1. The codes in categories ________________ and _________________ distinguish between uncomplicated cases and those in acute exacerbation.

2. An acute exacerbation is not equivalent to an infection superimposed on a chronic condition, though an exacerbation may be triggered by an infection.

   a. True
   b. False

3. Codes J96.0 and J96.2 may be assigned as a principal diagnosis when it is

   ____

   ____

   ____

4. Respiratory failure may be listed as a _______________________________ if it occurs after admission, or if it is present on admission, but does not meet the definition of principal diagnosis.

5. When a patient is admitted with respiratory failure and another acute condition, the principal diagnosis will not ____

6. If both the respiratory failure and the other acute condition are equally responsible for occasioning the admission to the hospital, and there are no chapter-specific sequencing rules, the guideline regarding two or more diagnoses that equally meet the definition for principal diagnosis may be applied in these situations.

   a. True
   b. False

7. If the documentation is not clear as to whether acute respiratory failure and another condition are equally responsible for occasioning the admission, the coder should____

8. Code only confirmed cases of influenza due to certain identified influenza viruses and due to other identified influenza virus.

    a. True
    b. False

9. Confirmation does require documentation of positive laboratory testing specific for avian, other novel influenza, or other identified influenza virus.

    a. True
    b. False

10. If the provider records "suspected" or "possible" or "probable" avian influenza, or novel influenza, or other identified influenza, then the appropriate code from Category ______________should be assigned.

11. As with all procedural or postprocedural complications, code assignment is based on the provider's documentation of the relationship between the ___________________and the ___________________________

12. Code J95.851, Ventilator associated pneumonia, should be assigned only when the provider has documented ventilator associated pneumonia (VAP).

    a. True
    b. False

13. As it relates to the previous question, an additional code to identify the organism should also be assigned; do not assign an additional code from categories J12-J18 to identify the type of pneumonia.

    a. True
    b. False

14. Code J95.851 should not be assigned for cases where the patient has pneumonia and is on a mechanical ventilator and the provider has not specifically stated that the pneumonia is ventilator-associated pneumonia.

    a. True
    b. False

15.   If the documentation is unclear as to whether the patient has a pneumonia that is a complication attributable to the mechanical ventilator, query the provider.

    a.   True
    b.   False

16.   A patient may be admitted with one type of pneumonia (e.g., code J13, Pneumonia due to Streptococcus pneumonia) and subsequently develop VAP. In this instance, the principal diagnosis would be the appropriate code from

____

____

17.   As it relates to the previous question, code J95.851, Ventilator associated pneumonia, would be assigned as an additional diagnosis when the provider has also documented the presence of ventilator associated pneumonia.

    a.   True
    b.   False

18.   For patients presenting with condition(s) related to vaping, assign code U07.0, \ as the ___________________ diagnosis.

19.   For lung injury due to vaping, assign only code ________________.

20.   Associated respiratory signs and symptoms due to vaping, such as cough, shortness of breath, etc., are not coded separately, when a definitive diagnosis has been established.

    a.   True
    b.   False

Diseases of Skin and Subcutaneous Tissue (L00-L99)

1. Codes from category L89, Pressure ulcer, are combination codes that identify the site of the pressure ulcer as well as the _______________________________________

2. The ICD-10-CM classifies ulcer stages based on severity, which is designated by:

    a. ____

    b. ____

    c. ____

3. Assign as many codes from Category L89 as needed to ____________ all the pressure ulcers the patient has, if applicable.

4. Assignment of the code for the unstageable pressure ulcer should be based on should be on clinical documentation.

    a. True
    b. False

5. When there is no documentation regarding the stage of the pressure ulcer, assign a code for ____

6. Assignment of the pressure ulcer stage code should be guided by clinical documentation of the ____

    ____

7. No code is assigned if the documentation states that pressure ulcer is completely healed.

    a. True
    b. False

8. Pressure ulcers described as ____________ should be assigned the appropriate pressure ulcer stage code based on the documentation in the medical record.

9. If the documentation does not provide information about the stage of the healing pressure, assign ____

10. If the documentation is unclear as to whether the patient has a current (new) pressure ulcer or if the patient is being treated for a healing pressure ulcer, query the provider.

    a. True
    b. False

11. For ulcers that were _______________ on admission but healed at the time of discharge, assign the code for the site and stage of the pressure ulcer at the time of admission.

12. If a patient is admitted with a pressure ulcer at one stage and it progresses to a higher stage, two separate codes should be assigned:

    a. ____

    b. ____

13. For pressure-induced deep tissue damage or deep tissue pressure injury, assign only the appropriate code for pressure-induced deep tissue damage (L89.--6).

    a. True
    b. False

14. No code is assigned if the documentation states that the non-pressure ulcer is completely _________________ at the time of admission.

15. Non-pressure ulcers described as _______________ should be assigned the appropriate non-pressure ulcer code based on the documentation in the medical record.

16. If the documentation does not provide information about the _____________ of the healing non-pressure ulcer, assign the appropriate code for unspecified severity.

17. If the documentation is unclear as to whether the patient has a current (new) non-pressure ulcer or if the patient is being treated for a healing non-pressure ulcer, _________________ the provider.

18. For ulcers that were present on admission but healed at the time of discharge, assign the code for the site and severity of the non-pressure ulcer at the time of admission.

    a.   True
    b.   False

19. If a patient is admitted to an inpatient hospital with a non-pressure ulcer at one severity level and it progresses to a higher severity level, two separate codes should be assigned:

    a.   ____

    b.   ____

Diseases of Musculoskeletal System and Connective Tissue (M00-M99)

1.   All of the codes within Chapter 13 have site and laterality designations.

    a.   True
    b.   False

2.   The site represents the _______________________, _____________________
    or the _______________________ involved.

3.   Though the portion of the bone affected may be at the joint, the site designation
    will be the bone, not the joint.

    a.   True
    b.   False

4.   Recurrent bone, joint or muscle conditions are also usually found in Chapter
    ________________. Any current, acute injury should be coded to the appropriate
    injury code from ____________________

5.   7th character A is for use as long as the patient is receiving active treatment for
    the fracture.

    a.   True
    b.   False

6.   7th character, D is to be used for encounters after the patient has completed
    active treatment for the fracture and is receiving routine care for the fracture
    during the healing or recovery phase.

    a.   True
    b.   False

7.   Care for complications of surgical treatment for fracture repairs during the
    healing or recovery phase should be coded with ______________________________

    ____

8.   Osteoporosis is a systemic condition, meaning that all bones of the musculoskeletal system are affected; therefore, site is not a component of the

____

9.   Category M81, Osteoporosis without current pathological fracture, is for use for patients with osteoporosis who do not currently have a ______________ fracture due to the osteoporosis, even if they have had a fracture in the past.

10.   For patients with a history of osteoporosis fractures, status code ______________ should follow the code from M81.

11.   Category M80, Osteoporosis with current pathologic fracture, is for patients who have a current ______________ fracture at the time of an encounter.

12.   The codes under M80 identify the ___________________ of the fracture.

13.   A code from category __________, not a traumatic fracture code, should be used for any patient with known osteoporosis who suffers a fracture, even if the patient had a minor fall or trauma, if that fall or trauma would not usually break a normal, healthy bone.

Diseases of Genitourinary System (N00-N99)

1. ICD-10-CM classifies chronic kidney disease (CKD) based on severity, which is designated by stages _______ to _________.

2. Stage 2, code N18.2, equates to ____

3. Stage 3, code N18.3, equates to ____

4. Stage 4, code N18.4, equates to ____

5. Code _________, End stage renal disease (ESRD), is assigned when the provider has documented end-stage renal disease (ESRD).

6. If both a stage of CKD and ESRD are documented, assign code _______________

7. Patients who have undergone kidney transplant may still have some form of CKD, because ____

   ____

8. Based on the previous question, the coder would assign the appropriate N18 code for the patient's stage of CKD and code ________________________________.

9. If the documentation is unclear as to whether the patient has a complication of the transplant, the coder should ____

10. The sequencing of the CKD code in relationship to codes for other contributing conditions is based on the conventions in the_______________________________.

Pregnancy, Childbirth, and the Puerperium (O00-O9A)

1. Chapter 15, codes in the range O00-O9A, Pregnancy, childbirth and the puerperium, do not have sequencing priority over chapters.

    a. True
    b. False

2. Should the provider document that the pregnancy is incidental to the encounter, then code ___________________ should be used in place of any chapter 15 codes.

3. Chapter 15 may be assigned to both maternal and newborn records.

    a. True
    b. False

4. The majority of codes in Chapter 15 have a final character indicating the

    ____

5. Assignment of the final character for trimester should be based on the provider's documentation of the trimester (or number of weeks) for the current admission/encounter.

    a. True
    b. False

6. Whenever delivery occurs during the current admission, and there is an "in childbirth" option for the obstetric complication being coded, the "in childbirth" code should not be assigned.

    a. True
    b. False

7. In instances when a patient is admitted to a hospital for complications of pregnancy during one trimester and remains in the hospital into a subsequent trimester, the trimester character for the ___________________________
    should be assigned on the basis of the trimester when the complication developed, not the trimester of the discharge.

8. If the condition developed prior to the current admission/encounter or represents a pre-existing condition, the trimester character _________________________

    ____

    ____

9. The "unspecified trimester" code should rarely be used, such as when the documentation in the record is insufficient to determine the trimester and it is not possible to obtain clarification.

    a. True
    b. False

10. Where applicable, a 7th character is to be assigned for certain categories (O31, O32, O33.3 - O33.6, O35, O36, O40, O41, O60.1, O60.2, O64, and O69) to identify the fetus for which the complication code applies. Assign 7th character "0":

    a. ____

    b. ____

        ____

    c. ____

        ____

11. In ICD-10-CM, ___________________ weeks of gestation refers to full weeks.

12. For routine outpatient prenatal visits when no complications are present, which code should be used? ____

13. Codes from Category O09, Supervision of high-risk pregnancy, are intended for use only during the prenatal period.

    a. True
    b. False

14.   For complications during the ____________ or _______________ episode as a result of a high-risk pregnancy, assign the applicable complication codes from Chapter 15.

15.   If there are no complications during the labor or delivery episode, assign code ____________.

16.   For routine prenatal outpatient visits for patients with ____________ pregnancies, a code from category O09, Supervision of high-risk pregnancy, should be used as the first-listed diagnosis.

17.   In episodes when no delivery occurs, the principal diagnosis should correspond to the principal complication of the pregnancy which necessitated the encounter; should more than one complication exist, all of which are treated or monitored, any of the complication codes may be sequenced _______________.

18.   When an obstetric patient is admitted and delivers during that admission, the condition that prompted the admission should be ____________ as the principal diagnosis.

19.   If multiple conditions prompted the admission, sequence the one most related to the delivery as the principal diagnosis; a code for any complication of the delivery should be assigned as an ____________ diagnosis.

20.   In cases of ____________ delivery, if the patient was admitted with a condition that resulted in the performance of a cesarean procedure that condition should be selected as the principal diagnosis.

21.   If the reason for the admission was __________ to the condition resulting in the cesarean delivery, the condition related to the reason for the admission should be selected as the principal diagnosis.

22.   A code from category Z37, Outcome of delivery, should be included on every maternal _______________ when a delivery has occurred.

23.   When assigning codes from Chapter 15, it is important to assess if a condition was pre-existing prior to pregnancy or developed during or due to the pregnancy in order to assign the correct code.

    a.   True
    b.   False

24.   It is acceptable to use codes specifically for the puerperium with codes complicating pregnancy and childbirth if a condition arises postpartum during the delivery encounter.

    a.   True
    b.   False

25.   When assigning one of the O10 codes that includes hypertensive heart disease or hypertensive chronic kidney disease, it is necessary to add a _______________ code from the appropriate hypertension category to specify the type of heart failure or chronic kidney disease.

26.   Codes from categories O35, Maternal care for known or suspected fetal abnormality and damage, and O36, Maternal care for other fetal problems, are assigned only when the fetal condition is actually responsible for modifying the management of the mother, i.e., by requiring diagnostic studies, additional observation, special care, or termination of pregnancy.

    a.   True
    b.   False

27.   The fact that the fetal condition exists does justify assigning a code from this series to the mother's record.

    a.   True
    b.   False

28.   In cases when surgery is performed on the fetus, a diagnosis from Category O35, Maternal care for known or suspected fetal abnormality and damage, should be assigned identifying the ____________ condition.

29.   No code from Chapter 16, the Perinatal codes, should be used on the mother's record to identify fetal conditions.

    a.   True
    b.   False

30. During pregnancy, childbirth, or the puerperium, a patient admitted because of an HIV-related illness should be coded with a principal diagnosis of ___________, followed by the codes for the ___________________ illness (es).

31. Patients with asymptomatic HIV infection status admitted during pregnancy, childbirth or the puerperium, assign codes____

32. Pregnant women who are diabetic should be assigned which codes?

    First listed____

    Second____

33. No other code from category O24, Diabetes mellitus in pregnancy, childbirth, and the puerperium, should be used with a code from O24.4

    a. True
    b. False

34. The codes under subcategory O24.4 include:

    a. ____

    b. ____

    c. ____

35. If a patient with gestational diabetes is treated with both diet and insulin, only the code for insulin-controlled is required.

    a. True
    b. False

36. An abnormal glucose tolerance in pregnancy is not assigned a code from subcategory O99.81, Abnormal glucose complicating pregnancy, childbirth, and the puerperium.

    a. True
    b. False

37.   When assigning a chapter 15 code for sepsis complicating abortion, pregnancy, childbirth, and the puerperium, a code for the specific type of _________________ should be assigned as an additional diagnosis.

38.   If severe sepsis is present, a code from subcategory R65.2, Severe sepsis, and code(s) for associated organ dysfunction(s) _________________________________

____

39.   Code O85, Puerperal sepsis, should be assigned with a secondary code to identify

____

40.   A code from category A40, Streptococcal sepsis, or A41, Other sepsis, should not be used for puerperal sepsis.

   a.   True
   b.   False

41.   Codes under subcategory O99.31, Alcohol use complicating pregnancy, childbirth, and the puerperium, should be assigned for any pregnancy case when a mother uses alcohol during the pregnancy or postpartum; a secondary code from category ________________, Alcohol related disorders, should also be assigned to identify manifestations of the alcohol use.

42.   Codes under subcategory O99.33, Smoking (tobacco) complicating pregnancy, childbirth, and the puerperium, should be assigned for any pregnancy case when a mother uses any type of tobacco product during the pregnancy or postpartum; a secondary code from category F17, Nicotine dependence, should not be assigned to identify the type of nicotine dependence.

43.   Codes under subcategory O99.32, Drug use complicating pregnancy, childbirth, and the puerperium, should be assigned for any pregnancy case when a mother uses drugs during the pregnancy or postpartum. This can involve illegal drugs, or inappropriate use or abuse of prescription drugs; secondary code(s) from categories _____________________ and ___________________ should also be assigned to identify manifestations of the drug use.

44. A code from subcategory O9A.2, Injury, poisoning and certain other consequences of external causes complicating pregnancy, childbirth, and the puerperium, should be sequenced first, followed by the appropriate injury, poisoning, toxic effect, adverse effect or underdosing code, and then the additional code(s) that specifies the condition caused by the poisoning, toxic effect, adverse effect or underdosing.

    a. True
    b. False

45. What are the conditions that must be met in order to assign code O80, Normal delivery?

    a. ____

    b. ____

    c. ____

46. Additional codes from other chapters may be used with code O80 if they are not related to or are in any way complicating the pregnancy.

    a. True
    b. False

47. Code O80 may be used if the patient ________________________________

    ____

    ____

    ____

48. What is the only code that is appropriate for use with code O80? ____________

49. The postpartum period begins ________________________________

    ____

    ____

50. The peripartum period is defined as the last ______________ of pregnancy to ______ months postpartum.

51. What is the definition of a postpartum complication?

    ____

    ____

52. Chapter 15 codes can be used to describe a pregnancy related complication after the six-week period.

    a. True
    b. False

53. When the mother delivers outside the hospital prior to admission and is admitted for routine postpartum care and no complications are noted, which code should be assigned as the principal diagnosis? _______________________________________

54. Code O90.3 may be diagnosed in the third trimester and continue to progress months after delivery.

    a. True
    b. False

55. Code O90.3 is only for use when _______________________________________

    ____

    ____

56. Code O94, Sequelae of complication of pregnancy, childbirth and the puerperium is for use in those cases when an _______________________________________

    ____

    ____

    ____

57.   When can code O94 be used? _______________________________________

____

58.   How is code O94 sequenced? _______________________________________

____

59.   When an attempted termination of pregnancy results in a liveborn infant, which codes are used?

a. First-listed____

b. Secondary ____

60.   Subsequent encounters for retained products of conception following a spontaneous or elective termination of pregnancy are assigned the appropriate code from

a. First-listed____

b. Secondary ____

c. Tertiary ____

61.   If the patient has a specific complication associated with the spontaneous abortion or elective termination of pregnancy in addition to retained products of conception, assign the appropriate complication in category O03 or O07 instead of code O03.4 or O07.4.

a.   True
b.   False

62.   Codes from Chapter 15 may be used as additional codes to identify any documented complications of the pregnancy in conjunction with codes in categories _________________, _________________and _________________.

63.   For hemorrhage post elective abortion, assign code ____________________.

64.   For suspected or confirmed cases of abuse of a pregnant patient, a code(s) from subcategories O9A.3, Physical abuse complicating pregnancy, childbirth, and the puerperium, O9A.4, Sexual abuse complicating pregnancy, childbirth, and the puerperium, and O9A.5, Psychological abuse complicating pregnancy, childbirth, and the puerperium, should be sequenced second.

    a.   True
    b.   False

65.   During pregnancy, childbirth or the puerperium, when COVID-19 is the reason for admission/encounter, code __________________ should be sequenced as the principal/first-listed diagnosis, and code U07.1, COVID-19, and the appropriate codes for associated manifestation(s) should be assigned as additional diagnoses.

66.   If the reason for admission/encounter is unrelated to COVID-19 but the patient tests positive for COVID-19 during the admission/encounter, the appropriate code for the reason for admission/encounter should be sequenced as the principal/first-listed diagnosis, and codes __________________ and __________________ as well as the appropriate codes for associated COVID-19 manifestations, should be assigned as additional diagnoses.

Newborn (Perinatal) Guidelines (P00-P96)

1. For coding and reporting purposes the perinatal period is defined as before _______ through the _______ day following birth.

2. Chapter 16 codes can be used on maternal records.

    a. True
    b. False

3. Chapter 16 codes may be used throughout the life of the patient if the condition is still present.

    a. True
    b. False

4. When coding the birth episode in a newborn, assign a code from category Z38 as secondary diagnosis.

    a. True
    b. False

5. A code from category Z38 is assigned only ___________, to a newborn at the time of birth.

6. If a newborn is transferred to another institution, a code from category Z38 should not be used at the receiving hospital.

    a. True
    b. False

7. A code from category Z38 is used only on the newborn record and not on the mother's record.

    a. True
    b. False

8.   Codes from other chapters may be used with codes from chapter 16 if the codes from the other chapters provide more specific ________________.

9.   If the reason for the encounter is a perinatal condition, the code from chapter 16 is sequenced first.

    a.   True
    b.   False

10.   Should a condition originate in the perinatal period, and continue throughout the life of the patient, the perinatal code should continue to be used regardless of the patient's age.

    a.   True
    b.   False

11.   If a newborn has a condition that may be either due to the birth process or community acquired, and the documentation does not indicate which it is, the default is ____

____

____

12.   A condition is clinically significant if it requires:

    a.   ____

    b.   ____

    c.   ____

    d.   ____

    e.   ____

    f.   ____

____

13. Codes should be assigned for conditions that have been specified by the provider as having implications for future health care needs.

    a. True
    b. False

14. Assign a code from category ____________, Observation and evaluation of newborns and infants for suspected diseases and conditions ruled out, to identify those instances when a healthy newborn is evaluated for a suspected condition/disease that is determined after study not to be present.

15. Do not use a code from category Z05 when the patient is documented to have signs or symptoms of a suspected problem; in such cases code the sign or symptom.

    a. True
    b. False

16. A code from category Z05 may also be assigned as a principal or first-listed code for readmissions or encounters when the code from category ________ code no longer applies.

17. Codes from category Z05 are for use only for healthy newborns and infants for which no condition after study is found to be present.

    a. True
    b. False

18. A code from category Z05 is to be used as a ________________ code after the code from category Z38, Liveborn infants according to place of birth and type of delivery.

19. Do not assign codes for conditions that require treatment or further investigation, prolong the length of stay, or require resource utilization.

    a. True
    b. False

20. Assign codes for conditions that have been specified by the provider as having implications for future health care needs.

    a.   True
    b.   False

21. A code for prematurity should not be assigned unless ______________________________

22. Assignment of codes in categories P05, Disorders of newborn related to slow fetal growth and fetal malnutrition, and P07, Disorders of newborn related to short gestation and low birth weight, not elsewhere classified, should be based on the recorded birth _______________and estimated __________________ age.

23. When both birth weight and gestational are available, two codes from category P07 should be assigned, with the code for _______________ __________________ sequenced before the code for gestational age.

24. Codes from category P07, Disorders of newborn related to short gestation and low birth weight, not elsewhere classified, are for use for a child or adult who had a low birth weight as a newborn and this is affecting the patient's current health status.

    a.   True
    b.   False

25. If a perinate is documented as having sepsis without documentation of congenital or community acquired, the default is congenital and a code from category ________ should be assigned.

26. If the P36 code does not include the causal organism, assign an additional code from category __________.

27. Code P95, stillbirth, is only for use institutions that maintain separate records for stillbirths.

    a.   True
    b.   False

28. For a newborn that tests positive for COVID-19, assign code U07.1, COVID-19, and the appropriate codes for associated manifestation(s) in neonates/newborns in the absence of documentation indicating a specific type of transmission.

    a.   True
    b.   False

29. For a newborn that tests positive for COVID-19 and the provider documents the condition was contracted in utero or during the birth process, assign codes P35.8, Other congenital viral diseases, and U07.1, COVID-19.

    a.   True
    b.   False

30. When coding the birth episode in a newborn record, the appropriate code from category Z38, Liveborn infants according to place of birth and type of delivery, should be assigned as the secondary diagnosis.

    a.   True
    b.   False

Congenital Malformations, Deformations/Chromosomal Abnormalities (Q00-Q99)

1. Assign code(s) from Categories Q00-Q99, Congenital malformations, deformations and chromosomal abnormalities when a malformation/deformation or _______________________________ is documented.

2. A malformation/deformation/or chromosomal abnormality may be the principal/first-listed diagnosis on a record or a secondary diagnosis.

    a. True
    b. False

3. When a malformation/deformation/or chromosomal abnormality does not have a ________________ code assignment, the coder should assign additional codes for any additional code(s) for any manifestations that may be present.

4. When the code assignment specifically identifies malformation/deformation/or chromosomal abnormality, manifestations that are an ________component of the anomaly should not be coded separately.

5. Codes from Chapter 17 may not be used throughout the life of the patient.

    a. True
    b. False

6. If a congenital malformation or deformity has been corrected, a personal history code should not be used to identify the history of the malformation and deformity.

    a. True
    b. False

7. Although present at birth, a malformation/deformation/or chromosomal abnormality may not be identified until ____.

8. Whenever the condition is diagnosed by the physician, it is appropriate to assign a code from codes Q00-Q99.

    a. True
    b. False

9. For the birth admission, the appropriate code from Category Z38 should be sequenced as the _____________________ diagnosis, followed by any congenital anomaly codes, Q00-Q99.

Symptoms, Signs and Abnormal Clinic and Laboratory Findings, NEC (R00-R99)

1.   Chapter 18 includes symptoms, signs, abnormal results of clinical or other investigative procedures, and ill-defined conditions regarding which no _____________________ classifiable elsewhere is recorded.

2.   Codes that describe symptoms and signs are acceptable for reporting purposes when a related definitive diagnosis has not been established by the provider.

    a.   True
    b.   False

3.   Codes for signs and symptoms _______ be reported in addition to a related definitive diagnosis when the sign or symptom is not routinely associated with that diagnosis.

4.   Signs or symptoms that are associated routinely with a disease process should not be assigned as additional codes, unless otherwise instructed by the classification.

    a.   True
    b.   False

5.   ICD-10-CM contains a number of combination codes that identify both the _____________________ diagnosis and _______________ symptoms of that diagnosis.

6.   _____________________ is for use for encounters when a patient has recently fallen and the reason for the fall is being investigated.

7.   _______________________ is for use when a patient has fallen in the past and is at risk for future falls.

8.   When appropriate, both codes R92.6 and Z91.81 may be assigned together.

    a.   True
    b.   False

9. The coma scale codes can be used in conjunction with traumatic brain injury codes, acute cerebrovascular disease or sequelae of cerebrovascular disease codes.

    a. True
    b. False

10. The coma scale codes should be ________________ after the diagnosis code(s).

11. Coma scale codes include a 7th character which indicates when the scale was recorded.

    a. True
    b. False

12. Assign code R40.24, Glasgow coma scale, total score, when only the total score is documented in the medical record and not the individual score(s).

    a. True
    b. False

13. When SIRS is documented with a noninfectious condition, and no subsequent infection is documented, the code for the underlying condition, such as an injury, should be assigned, followed by code ____________, Systemic inflammatory response syndrome (SIRS) of non-infectious origin without acute organ dysfunction, or code ____________, Systemic inflammatory response syndrome (SIRS) of non-infectious origin with acute organ dysfunction.

14. If an associated ______________________ is documented, the appropriate code(s) for the specific type of organ dysfunction(s) should be assigned in addition to code R65.11.

15. If acute organ dysfunction is documented, but it cannot be determined if the acute organ dysfunction is associated with SIRS or due to another condition, the provider should be ___________.

16. Code R99, is only for use in very limited situations when a patient who has already died is brought into an emergency department or other healthcare facility and is pronounced dead upon arrival. It also represents the discharge disposition of death.

    a. True
    b. False

17. The NIH stroke scale (NIHSS) codes (R29.7- -) can be used in _______________ with acute stroke codes (I63) to identify the patient's neurological status and the severity of the stroke.

18. The stroke scale codes should be sequenced _________ the acute stroke diagnosis code(s).

Injury, Poisoning and Certain Other Consequences of External Causes (S00-T88)

1.   Most categories in chapter 19 have a ______________ character requirement for each applicable code.

2.   Most categories in chapter 19 have three 7th character values, with the exception of fractures.

    a.   True
    b.   False

3.   Categories for traumatic fractures have ______________ 7th character values.

4.   While the patient may be seen by a new or different provider over the course of treatment for an injury, assignment of the 7th character is based on whether the patient is undergoing ______________treatment and not whether the provider is ______________ the patient for the first time.

5.   For complication codes, active treatment refers to treatment for the condition described by the code, even though it may be related to an earlier precipitating problem.

    a.   True
    b.   False

6.   7th character __________ initial encounter is used for each encounter where the patient is receiving active treatment.

7.   7th character __________ subsequent encounter is used for encounters after the patient has completed active treatment of the condition and is receiving routine care for the condition during the healing or recovery phase.

8.   The aftercare Z codes should not be used for aftercare for injuries, where 7th characters are provided to identify subsequent care.

    a.   True
    b.   False

9.   7th character _________ sequela is used for complications or conditions that arise as a direct result of a condition.

10.   When using 7th character "S", it is necessary to use both the __________________ code that precipitated the sequela and the code for the ___________________ itself.

11.   The 7th character "S" identifies the injury responsible for the sequela. The specific type of _________ is sequenced first, followed by the ____________ code.

12.   When coding injuries, assign separate codes for each injury unless a combination code is provided, in which case the combination code is assigned.

     a.   True
     b.   False

13.   Codes from category T07, unspecified multiple injuries should not be assigned in the ______________ setting unless information for a more specific code is not available.

14.   Traumatic injury codes (S00-T14.9) can be used for normal, healing surgical wounds or to identify complications of surgical wounds.

     a.   True
     b.   False

15.   The code for the most serious injury, as determined by the provider and the focus of the treatment, is sequenced first.

     a.   True
     b.   False

16.   Superficial injuries such as abrasions or contusions are ____________________ when associated with more severe injuries of the same site.

17.   When a primary injury results in minor damage to peripheral nerves or blood vessels, the primary injury is sequenced second with additional code(s) for injuries to nerves and spinal cord.

     a.   True
     b.   False

18.   When the _______________ injury is to the blood vessels or nerves, that injury should be sequenced first.

19.   Injury codes from Chapter 19 should not be assigned for injuries that occur during, or as a result of, a medical intervention.

    a.   True
    b.   False

20.   Fractures of specified sites are coded _________________________________ by site in accordance with both the provisions within categories S02, S12, S22, S32, S42, S49, S52, S59, S62, S72, S79, S82, S89, S92 and the level of detail furnished by medical record content.

21.   A fracture not indicated as ___________ or ____________ should be coded to closed.

22.   A fracture not indicated whether ___________ or _______________ should be coded to displaced.

23.   __________________ fractures are coded using the appropriate 7th character extension for initial encounter (A, B, C) for each encounter where the patient is receiving active treatment for the fracture.

24.   The appropriate 7th character for ________________ encounter should also be assigned for a patient who delayed seeking treatment for the fracture or nonunion.

25.   Fractures are coded using the appropriate 7th character for subsequent care for encounters after the patient has completed active treatment of the fracture and is receiving routine care for the fracture during the healing or recovery phase.

    a.   True
    b.   False

26.   Care for complications of surgical treatment for fracture repairs during the healing or recovery phase should be coded with the appropriate complication codes.

    a.   True
    b.   False

27. Care of complications of fractures should be reported with the appropriate 7th character extensions for subsequent care with nonunion (K, M, N,) or subsequent care with malunion (P, Q, R).

    a. True
    b. False

28. The appropriate _____ character for initial encounter should also be assigned for a patient who delayed seeking treatment for the fracture or nonunion.

29. The open fracture designations in the assignment of the 7th character for fractures of the forearm, femur and lower leg, including ankle are based on the _________________ open fracture classification.

30. When the Gustilo classification type is not specified for an open fracture, the 7th character for open fracture type I or II should be assigned (B, E, H, M, Q).

    a. True
    b. False

31. A code from category M80, not a traumatic fracture code, should be used for any patient with known osteoporosis who suffers a fracture, even if the patient had a minor fall or trauma, if that fall or trauma would not usually break a normal, healthy bone.

    a. True
    b. False

32. The aftercare Z codes should not be used for aftercare for traumatic fractures. For aftercare of a traumatic fracture, assign the acute fracture code with the appropriate __________ character.

33. Multiple fractures are sequenced in accordance with the ______________ of the fracture.

34. The ICD-10-CM makes a distinction between burns and corrosions.

    a. True
    b. False

35.   The ___________________________codes are for thermal burns, except sunburns, that come from a heat source, electricity and radiation.

36.   Corrosions are burns due to ________________.

37.   The guidelines are not the same for burns and corrosions.

      a.   True
      b.   False

38.   Current burns are classified by ________________, ___________________and by _______________________________

39.   Burns are classified by depth as follows:

      a.   ____

      b.   ____

      c.   ____

40.   Burns of the eye and internal organs are classified by _________________, but not by degree.

41.   Sequence _________________the code that reflects the highest degree of burn when more than one burn is present.

42.   When the reason for the admission or encounter is for treatment of external multiple burns, sequence _________________ the code that reflects the burn of the highest degree.

43.   When a patient has both internal and external burns, the circumstances of ___________________ govern the selection of the principal or first-listed diagnosis.

44.   When a patient is admitted for burn injuries and other related conditions such as smoke inhalation and/or respiratory failure, the circumstances of the admission do not govern the selection of the principal or first-listed diagnosis.

      a.   True
      b.   False

45. Burns of the same local site but of different degrees should be classified to the subcategory identifying the ______________ degree recorded in the diagnosis.

46. Non-healing burns are coded as ______________ burns.

47. Necrosis of burned skin should be coded as non-healed burn.

    a. True
    b. False

48. For any documented infected burn site, use an ________________ code for the infection.

49. When coding burns, assign ________________ codes for each burn site.

50. Category T30, Burn and corrosion, body region unspecified is ________________ vague and should ____________ be used.

51. Coders should assign codes T31 (burns classified according to extent of body surface burned) or T32 (Corrosions classified according to extent of body surface involved) when the site of the burn is not specified or when there is a need for additional data.

    a. True
    b. False

52. It is advisable to use category T31 as additional coding when needed to provide data for evaluating ____________________, such as that needed by burn units.

53. It is also advisable to use category T31 as an additional code for reporting purposes when there is mention of a ____________ burn involving 20 percent or more of the body surface.

54. Category T31 and T32 are based on the classic _________ of nines in estimating body surface involved.

55. Encounters for treatment of the sequelas of burns or corrosions should be coded with the 7th character of _________.

56. When appropriate, both a code for a current burn or corrosion with 7th character extension _________ or __________ and a burn or corrosion code with extension "S" may be assigned on the same record (when both a current burn and sequelae of an old burn exist).

57. An _________________________________ code should be used with burns and corrosions to identify the   source and intent of the burn, as well as the place where it occurred.

58. Codes in categories T36-T65 are __________________ codes that include the substance that was taken as well as the intent.

59. When using categories T36-T65 an additional code is needed to show the external cause of the poisoning, toxic effects, adverse effects and underdosing codes.

    a.   True
    b.   False

60. Coders may code directly from the Table of Drugs and Chemicals and there is no need to verify the code in the tabular list.

    a.   True
    b.   False

61. Use as many codes as necessary to describe completely all drugs, medicinal or biological substances.

    a.   True
    b.   False

62. If the same code would describe the causative agent for more than one adverse reaction, poisoning, toxic effect or underdosing, assign the code twice.

    a.   True
    b.   False

63. If two or more drugs, medicinal or biological substances are reported, code each individually unless a ____________________________is listed in the Table of Drugs and Chemicals.

64. When coding an adverse effect of a drug that has been correctly prescribed and administered, assign codes:

    a. ____

    b. ____

65. When coding a poisoning or reaction to the improper use of a medication, first assign code from categories: _______-________.

66. If the intent of the poisoning is unknown or unspecified, code the intent as ____________________ intent.

67. The undetermined intent is only for use if the documentation in the record specifies that the intent cannot be determined.

    a. True
    b. False

68. If there is also a diagnosis of abuse or dependence of a substance, the abuse or dependence is assigned as ____

69. Codes for underdosing should never be assigned as ____________ or first-listed.

70. If a patient has a ___________ or exacerbation of the medical condition for which the drug is prescribed because of the reduction in dose, then the medical condition itself should be coded.

71. Noncompliance or complication of care codes are to be used with an underdosing code to indicate the intent, if known.

    a. True
    b. False

72. When a harmful substance is ingested or comes in contact with a person, this is classified as a _____________ effect.

73. Toxic effect codes (T51-T65) have an associated intent, which can be classified in four ways which are:

    a. ____

    b. ____

    c. ____

    d. ____

74. Sequence first the appropriate code from categories T74. - (Adult and child abuse, neglect and other maltreatment, confirmed) or T76. - (Adult and child abuse, neglect and other maltreatment, suspected) for abuse, neglect and other maltreatment, followed by any accompanying mental health or injury codes.

    a. True
    b. False

75. If the documentation in the medical record states abuse or neglect it is coded as confirmed ________________. It is coded as suspected if it is documented as suspected __________________.

76. For cases of confirmed abuse or neglect an external cause code from the assault section ______________________should be added to identify the cause of any physical injuries.

77. A ________________________________ should be added when the perpetrator of the abuse is known.

78. If a suspected case of abuse, neglect or mistreatment is ruled out during an encounter code Z04.71 (encounter for examination and observation following alleged physical adult abuse, ruled out), or code Z04.72 (encounter for examination and observation following alleged child physical abuse, ruled out) should be used, not a code from T76.

    a. True
    b. False

79. If a suspected case of alleged rape or sexual abuse is ruled out during an encounter code Z04.41 (encounter for examination and observation following alleged adult rape), or code Z04.42 (encounter for examination and observation following alleged child rape) should be used, not a code from T76.

    a. True
    b. False

80. If a suspected case of forced sexual exploitation or forced labor exploitation is ruled out during an encounter, code _______________, Encounter for examination and observation of victim following forced sexual exploitation, or code ____________, Encounter for examination and observation of victim following forced labor exploitation, should be used, not a code from T76.

81. _________________associated with devices, implants or grafts left in a surgical site (for example painful hip prosthesis) is assigned to the appropriate code(s) found in Chapter 19, Injury, poisoning, and certain other consequences of external causes.

82. Specific codes for pain due to medical devices are found in the________ code section of the ICD-10-CM; use additional code(s) from category ________ to identify acute or chronic pain due to presence of the device, implant or graft (G89.19 or G89.28)

83. Codes under Category T86 are for use for both ________________ and rejection of transplanted organ.

84. A transplant complication code is only assigned if the complication affects the function ____

85. Two codes are required to fully describe a transplant complication:

    a. ____

    b. ____

86. Pre-existing conditions or conditions that develop after the transplant are not coded as complications unless they __________ the function of the transplanted organs.

87. Code ______________ should be assigned for documented complications of a kidney transplant.

88. Code T86.1- should not be assigned for post ______________ transplant patients who have CKD unless a transplant complication such as transplant failure or rejection is documented.

89. If the documentation is unclear as to whether the patient has a complication of the transplant, the coder should ____

90. Conditions that affect the function of the transplanted kidney, other than CKD, should be assigned the following codes:

    a. ____

    b. ____

91. As with certain other T codes, some of the complications of care codes have the external cause included in the code.
    a.   True
    b.   False

92. Intraoperative and postprocedural complication codes are found within the body system chapters with codes specific to the organs and structures of that body system. These codes should be sequenced first, followed by a code(s) for the specific complication, if applicable.

    a.   True
    b.   False

93. Complication codes from the body system chapters should be assigned for intraoperative and postprocedural complications unless the complication is specifically indexed to a T code in chapter 19.

    a.   True
    b.   False

External Causes of Morbidity (V01-Y99)

1. The external causes of morbidity codes are never sequenced as the first-listed or principal diagnosis.

    a.   True
    b.   False

2. External cause codes are not intended to provide data for injury research and evaluation of injury prevention strategies.

    a.   True
    b.   False

3. External cause codes capture:

    a.   ____

    b.   ____

    c.   ____

    d.   ____

    e.   ____

4. An external cause code may be used with any code in the range of ____ classification that is a health condition due to an external cause.

5. Assign the external cause code, without the appropriate 7th character (initial encounter, subsequent encounter or sequela) for each encounter for which the injury or condition is being treated.

    a.   True
    b.   False

6. Most categories in chapter 20 have a _______ character requirement for each applicable code; most categories in this chapter have three 7th character values: _______, initial encounter, _______, subsequent encounter and ______, sequela.

7.   While the patient may be seen by a new or different provider over the course of treatment for an injury or condition, assignment of the 7th character for external cause should _______________ the 7th character of the code assigned for the associated injury or condition for the encounter.

8.   Use the _______ range of external cause codes to completely describe the cause, the intent, the place of occurrence, and if applicable, the activity of the patient at the time of the event, and the patient's status, for all injuries, and other health conditions due to an external cause.

9.   Assign as many external cause codes as necessary to fully ___________________

____

10.   If only one external code can be recorded, assign the code most related to the

____

11.   The selection of the appropriate external cause code is guided by the ______________________________ External Causes and by Inclusion and Exclusion notes in the Tabular List.

12.   An external cause code can never be reported as principal or first-listed diagnosis.

    a.   True
    b.   False

13.   The combination external cause code used should not correspond to the sequence of events regardless of which caused the most serious injury.

    a.   True
    b.   False

14.   An external cause code from Chapter 20 is needed if the external cause and intent are included in a code from another chapter.

    a.   True
    b.   False

15. Codes from category Y92 are secondary codes for use after other external cause codes to identify the location ____

    ____

16. A place of occurrence code is used only once, at the initial encounter for treatment.

    a.   True
    b.   False

17. 7th characters are used for Y92.

    a.   True
    b.   False

18. Y92.9 can be used if the place of occurrence is not stated.

    a.   True
    b.   False

19. Assign a code from category ___________________ to describe the activity of the patient at the time the injury or other health condition occurred.

20. An activity code may be reported once, at the initial encounter for treatment.

    a.   True
    b.   False

21. Only one code from Y93 should be recorded on a medical record.

    a.   True
    b.   False

22. The activity codes are applicable to poisonings, adverse effects, misadventures or sequelas.

    a.   True
    b.   False

23. Do not assign Y93.9, Unspecified activity, if the activity is not stated.

    a. True
    b. False

24. A code from category _______________ is appropriate for use with external cause and intent codes if identifying the activity provides additional information about the event.

25. When applicable, place of occurrence, activity, and external cause status codes are sequenced after ____

26. Regardless of the number of external cause codes assigned, there should be only one:

    a. ____

    b. ____

    c. ____

27. If the reporting format limits the number of external cause codes that can be used in reporting clinical data, report the code for the cause/intent most related to the ____

28. If the format permits capture of additional external cause codes, the ________/ __________including medical misadventures, of the additional events should be reported rather than the codes for place, activity, or external status.

29. If two or more events cause separate injuries, an external cause code should be assigned for each cause. The first-listed external cause code will be selected in the following order:

    a. External cause codes for _____________________________ take priority over all other external cause codes.

    b. External cause codes for _____________________________ take priority over all other external cause codes except child and adult abuse.

    c.   External cause codes for ________________________________ take priority over all other external cause codes except child and adult abuse and terrorism.

    d.   External cause codes for ______________________________ take priority over all other external cause codes except cataclysmic events, child and adult abuse and terrorism.

    e.   __________ and external cause status codes are assigned following all causal (intent) external cause codes.

    f.   The ___________________external cause code should correspond to the cause of the most serious diagnosis due to an assault, accident, or self-harm.

30.   Adult and child abuse, neglect and maltreatment are classified as ______________

31.   For confirmed cases of abuse, neglect and maltreatment, when the perpetrator is known a code from ____ should accompany any other assault codes.

32.   If the intent (accident, self-harm, assault) of the cause of an injury or other condition is unknown or unspecified, code the intent as_____________________

33.   All _______________ accident categories assume accidental intent.

34.   External cause codes for events of undetermined intent are only for use if the documentation in the record specifies that the intent cannot be determined.

    a.   True
    b.   False

35.   Sequelas are reported using the 7th character _________ for sequela; these codes _________________ be used with any report of a late effect or sequela resulting from a previous injury.

36.   A sequela external cause code should never be used with a related _____________ nature of injury code.

37.   Use a late effect external cause code for subsequent visits when a late effect of the initial injury is being _________________.

38. Do not use a sequela external cause code for subsequent visits for follow-up care of the injury when no late effect of the ______________ has been documented.

39. When the cause of an injury is identified by the FBI as terrorism, the first-listed external cause code should be a code from category____________________.

40. Where is the definition of terrorism employed by the FBI found in the ICD-10-CM? ____

41. More than one Y38 code may be assigned if the injury is the result of more than one mechanism of terrorism.

    a. True
    b. False

42. When the cause of an injury is suspected to be the result of terrorism a code from category ____________________ should not be assigned.

43. Suspected cases should be classified as ___________________.

44. Which code should be assigned for conditions occurring subsequent to the terrorist event? ____

45. It is not acceptable to assign code Y38.9 with another code from Y38 if there is an injury due to the initial terrorist event and an injury that is a subsequent result of the terrorist event.

    a. True
    b. False

46. A code from category Y99, External cause status, ______________ be assigned whenever any other external cause code is assigned for an encounter, including an Activity code.

47. Assign a code from category Y99 (external cause status) to indicate the ________ status of the person at the time the even occurred.

48. The status code indicates whether the event occurred during:

    a. ____

    b. ____

    c. ____

49. Assign a code from category Y99 (external cause status) when applicable, with other external cause codes.

    a. True
    b. False

50. The external cause status codes are not applicable to:

    a. ____

    b. ____

    c. ____

    d. ____

51. Do not assign a code from category Y99 if _______________________________ codes (cause, activity) are applicable for the encounter.

52. An external cause status code is used _________________, at the initial encounter for treatment.

53. Only one code from Y99 should be recorded on a medical record.

    a. True
    b. False

54. Do not assign code Y99.9, Unspecified external cause status, if the status is not stated.

    a. True
    b. False

Factors Influencing Health Status and Contact with Health Service (Z00-Z99)

1. Z codes are for use in any health care setting and may be used as either a first-listed (principal diagnosis code in the inpatient setting) or secondary code, depending on the circumstances of the encounter.

    a. True
    b. False

2. ___________ Z codes may only be used as first-listed or principal diagnosis.

3. Z codes can be used as procedure codes.

    a. True
    b. False

4. A _____________ procedure codes must accompany a Z code to describe any procedure performed.

5. Category ___________ indicates contact with, and suspected exposure to communicable diseases.

6. Category Z20 codes are for patients who do not show any sign or symptom of a disease but are _________________ to have been exposed to it by close personal contact with an infected individual or are in an area where a disease is epidemic.

7. Category ________ indicates contact with and suspected exposures hazardous to health.

8. Contact/exposure codes may be used as a _________________ code to explain an encounter for testing, or, more commonly, as a secondary code to identify a potential risk.

9. Code Z23 is for encounters for ____________________ and ____________________

10. ___________________codes are required to identify the actual administration of the injection and the type(s) of immunizations given.

11. Code Z23 may be used as a _________________ code if the inoculation is given as a routine part of preventive health care, such as a well-baby visit.

12. __________________codes indicate that a patient is either a carrier of a disease or has the sequelae or residual of a past disease or condition.

13. A status code is informative, because the status may affect the course of ________________ and its _____________________

14. A status code is distinct from a history code, as it indicates that the patient ____ longer has the condition.

15. A status code should be used with a diagnosis code from one of the body system chapters, if the diagnosis code includes the information provided by the status code.

    a. True
    b. False

16. For encounters for ______________ from a mechanical ventilator, assign a code from subcategory J96.1, Chronic respiratory failure, followed by code Z99.11, Dependence on respirator [ventilator] status.

17. Codes from category Z15 should not be used as principal or first-listed codes.

    a. True
    b. False

18. As it relates to the previous question, if the patient has the condition to which he/she is ______________, and that condition is the reason for the encounter, the code for the current condition should be sequenced first.

19. As it relates to Z15, if the patient is being seen for follow-up after completed treatment for this condition and the condition no longer exists, which codes should be assigned?

    a. ____

    b. ____

20. If the purpose of the encounter is genetic counseling associated with procreative management, code Z31.5, Encounter for genetic counseling, should be assigned as the first-listed code, followed by a code from category ______________.

21.   _________ indicates that a patient has a condition that is resistant to antimicrobial drug treatment; sequence the infection code first.

22.   ___________ indicates that a patient has tested positive for HIV but has manifested no signs or symptoms of the disease.

23.   ___________ indicates that a person harbors the specific organisms of a disease without manifest symptoms and is capable of transmitting the infection.

24.   Z33.1 is a _______________ code only for use when the pregnancy is in no way complicating the reason for the visit.

25.   _________ is used when it is documented by the provider that a patient is on do not resuscitate status at any time during the stay.

26.   Z68, body mass index codes should only be assigned as a secondary diagnosis code, when it meets the definition of a _______________ diagnosis.

27.   Code Z78.1, Physical restraint status, may be used when it is documented by the provider that a patient has been put in restraints during the current encounter.

    a.   True
    b.   False

28.   Codes in category Z79 indicate a patient's _______________ use of a prescribed drug for the long-term treatment of a condition for prophylactic use. Do not assign a code from category Z79 for ____________ being administered for a brief period of time to treat an acute illness or injury.

29.   Assign code ____________ Status post administration of tPA (rtPA) in a different facility within the last 24 hours prior to admission to current facility, as a secondary diagnosis when a patient is received by transfer into a facility and documentation indicates they were administered tissue plasminogen activator (tPA) within the last 24 hours prior to admission to the current facility.

30.   The appropriate code for the condition for which tPA was administered should be assigned first.

    a.   True
    b.   False

31.   There are two types of history Z codes, _________________ and _____________

32.   _________________history codes explain a patient's past medical condition that no longer exists and is not receiving any treatment, but that has the potential for recurrence, and therefore may require continued monitoring.

33.   _________________history codes are for use when a patient has a family member(s) who has had a particular disease that causes the patient to be at higher risk of also contracting the disease.

34.   _______________ history codes may be used in conjunction with follow-up codes and _______________history codes may be used in conjunction with screening codes to explain the need for a test or procedure.

35.   History codes are also acceptable on any medical record regardless of the reason for visit.

    a.   True
    b.   False

36.   A history of an illness, even if no longer _______________, is important information that may alter the type of treatment ordered.

37.   _______________________________ is the testing for disease or disease precursors in seemingly well individuals so that early detection and treatment can be provided for those who test positive for the disease.

38.   The testing of a person to rule out or confirm a suspected diagnosis because the patient has some sign or symptom is a _________________________________, not a screening.

39.   A screening code may be a _____________________________ code if the reason for the visit is specifically the screening exam. It may also be used as an additional code if the _________________ is done during an office visit for other health problems.

40.   A screening code is not necessary if the screening is _________________ to a routine examination.

41.   Should a condition be discovered during the screening then the code for the _________________ may be assigned as an additional diagnosis.

42. The Z code indicates that the screening exam is _____________; a procedure code is required to confirm that the screening was _________________.

43. Observation codes are used in _________ limited circumstances when a person is being observed for a suspected condition that is ruled out.

44. Observation codes are not for use if an _____________ or _____________________ or any signs or symptoms are present.

45. Observation codes are primarily to be used as principal/first-listed diagnosis.

    a.   True
    b.   False

46. An observation code may be assigned as a secondary diagnosis code when the patient is being observed for a condition that is ruled out and is _____________ to the principal/first-listed diagnosis.

47. When the principal diagnosis is required to be a code from category Z38, Liveborn infants according to place of birth and type of delivery, then a code from category Z05, Encounter for observation and evaluation of newborn for suspected diseases and conditions ruled out, is sequenced after the Z38 code. , additional codes may be used in addition to the observation code, but only if they are unrelated to the suspected condition being observed.

    a.   True
    b.   False

48. Codes from subcategory Z03.7 may either be used as _________________ or as an additional code assignment depending on the case; they are very use in very limited circumstances on a maternal record when an encounter is for a suspected maternal or fetal condition that is _____________out during that encounter.

49. Codes from subcategory Z03.7 may not be used when the condition is confirmed.

    a.   True
    b.   False

50. Additional codes may be used in conjunction with Z03.7 only if they are related to the suspected condition.

    a. True
    b. False

51. Aftercare visit codes cover situations when the ______________ treatment of a disease has been performed and the patient requires continued care during the healing or recovery phase, or for the long-term consequences of the disease.

52. The aftercare Z codes should not be used if treatment is directed at a current, acute disease.

    a. True
    b. False

53. The aftercare Z codes should also not be assigned for aftercare for injuries; for aftercare of an injury, assign the acute injury code with the appropriate _______ character.

54. The aftercare codes are generally ____________________ to explain the specific reason for the encounter.

55. An aftercare code may be used as an additional code when some type of aftercare is provided in addition to the ______________ for admission and no ________________ code is applicable.

56. Aftercare codes should be used in conjunction with other aftercare or diagnosis codes to provide better detail on the specifics of an aftercare encounter visit, unless otherwise ___________ by the classification.

57. Certain aftercare Z code categories need a secondary diagnosis to describe the resolving ____.

58. Status ______ codes may be used with aftercare Z codes to indicate the nature of the aftercare.

59. A _________ code should not be used when the aftercare code indicates the type of status.

60. The follow-up codes are used to explain continuing surveillance following completed treatment of a disease, condition, or injury; they imply that the condition has been __________ treated and no longer ____________.

61. Follow-up codes should not be confused with __________codes, or injury codes with a 7th character for subsequent encounter, that explain ongoing care of a healing condition or its sequelae.

62. Follow-up codes may be used in conjunction with history codes to provide the full picture of the healed condition and its treatment; the follow-up code is sequenced first, followed by the history code.

    a. True
    b. False

63. A follow-up code may be used to explain multiple visits, should a condition be found to have reoccurred on the follow-up visit, in this case the ________________ code for the condition should be assigned in place of the follow-up code.

64. Codes in category Z52 are used for self-donations of blood, not for cadaveric donations.

    a. True
    b. False

65. ________________ Z codes are used when a patient or family member receives assistance in the aftermath of an illness or injury, or when support is required in coping with family or social problems.

66. Z codes for pregnancy are for use in those circumstances when none of the problems or complications included in codes from the Obstetrics chapter exist.

    a. True
    b. False

67. Codes in category Z34, Encounter for supervision of normal pregnancy, are always first-listed and are _________ to be used with any other code from the OB chapter.

68. Codes in category Z3A, Weeks of gestation, may be assigned to provide __________________ information about the ________________.

69.   Category Z3A codes should not be assigned for pregnancies with abortive outcomes (categories O00-O08), elective termination of pregnancy (code Z33.2), nor for postpartum conditions, as category Z3A is not applicable to these conditions.

   a.   True
   b.   False

70.   The __________ of the admission should be used to determine weeks of gestation for inpatient admissions that encompass more than one gestational week

71.   The outcome of delivery, category Z37 should be included on all maternal delivery records.

   a.   True
   b.   False

72.   Codes in category __________ should not be used on the newborn record.

73.   Z codes for __________________ or procreative management and counseling should be included on an obstetric record either during the pregnancy or the postpartum stage, if applicable.

74.   Routine and administrative examination Z codes allow for the description of encounters for routine examinations; these codes are not to be used if the examination is for diagnosis of a suspected condition or for treatment purposes.

   a.   True
   b.   False

75.   During a routine exam, should a diagnosis or condition be discovered, it should be coded as an additional code.

   a.   True
   b.   False

76.   Pre-existing and chronic conditions and history codes may also be included as additional codes as long as the examination is for ________________________ purposes and not focused on any particular condition.

77. Some of the codes for routine health examinations distinguish between "with" and "without" abnormal findings, code assignment depends on the information that is known at the _____________ of the encounter.

78. When assigning a code for "with abnormal findings," additional code(s) should be assigned to _____________ the specific abnormal findings.

79. Pre-operative examinations and pre-procedural laboratory examination Z codes are for use only in those situations when a patient is being cleared for a procedure or surgery and no treatment is given.

    a.   True
    b.   False

80. For encounters specifically for prophylactic removal of an organ (such as prophylactic removal of breasts due to a genetic susceptibility to cancer or a family history of cancer), which two codes should be used?

    a. ____

    b. ____

81. If the patient has a malignancy of one site and is having prophylactic removal at another site to prevent either a new primary malignancy or metastatic disease, a code for the malignancy should also be assigned in addition to subcategory code Z40, Encounter for prophylactic surgery for risk factors related to malignant neoplasms.

    a.   True
    b.   False

82. A _____________________code should not be assigned if the patient is having organ removal for treatment of a malignancy.

83. Certain Z codes are so non-specific, or potentially redundant with other codes in the classification, that there can be little justification for their use in the _____________________ setting; their use in the _____________________ setting should be limited to those instances when there is no further documentation to permit _____________________________________.

84. Social determinants of health (SDOH) codes describing social problems, conditions, or risk factors that influence a patient's health should be assigned when this information is ___________________ in the patient's medical record.

85. Assign as _____________ SDOH codes as are necessary to describe all of the social problems, conditions, or risk factors documented during the current episode of care.

Chapter 3-Selection of Principal and Secondary Diagnosis

1.   What is the definition of principal diagnosis?

____

____

____

____

2.   The UHDDS definitions are used by hospitals to report outpatient data elements in a standardized manner.

    a.   True
    b.   False

3.   In determining the principal diagnosis, coding conventions in the ICD-10-CM, the Tabular list and Alphabetic Index take precedence over the official coding guidelines.

    a.   True
    b.   False

4.   The importance of consistent, complete documentation in the medical record cannot be overemphasized; without such documentation the _________________ of all coding guidelines is a difficult, if not _____________________ task.

5.   Codes for symptoms, signs and ill-defined conditions from Chapter 18 are not meant to be used as principal diagnosis when a definitive diagnosis has been established.

    a.   True
    b.   False

6.   When there are two or more interrelated conditions potentially meeting the definition of principal diagnosis, which condition should be sequenced first?

____

____

____

____

____

7.   In the unusual instance when two or more diagnoses equally meet the criteria for principal diagnosis as determined by the circumstances of admission, diagnostic workup and/or therapy provided, and the Alphabetical Index, Tabular List, or another coding guideline does not provide sequencing direction, any one of the ___________________ may be sequenced first.

8.   What is the rule when two or more contrasting or comparative diagnoses are documented as "either/or"?

____

____

____

____

9.   How does the fact that the original treatment plan was not carried out influence the principal diagnosis assignment?

____

____

____

____

10. What is used as the principal diagnosis to identify a complication resulting from surgery or medical care?

     ____

11. If the complication is classified to the T80-T88 series and the code lacks the necessary specificity in describing the complication, an additional code for the specific complication should be assigned.

     a. True
     b. False

12. What is the rule for "uncertain diagnosis" as it relates to the principal diagnosis assignment? ____

     ____

13. When a patient is admitted to an observation unit for a medical condition, which either worsens or does not improve, and is subsequently admitted as an inpatient at the same hospital for this same medical condition, what is the principal diagnosis?

     ____

     ____

14. When a patient is admitted to an observation unit to monitor a condition (or complication) that develops following outpatient surgery, and then is subsequently admitted as an inpatient at the same hospital, hospitals should apply the UHDDS definition of____.

15. When a patient receives surgery in the hospital's outpatient surgery department and is subsequently admitted for continuing inpatient care at the same hospital, what guidelines should be followed in selecting the principal diagnosis?

a. ____

____

____

____

____

b. ____

____

____

____

____

c. ____

____

____

____

16. When the purpose for the admission/encounter is rehabilitation, sequence first the code for the condition for which the service is being performed.

    a. True
    b. False

17. If the condition for which the rehabilitation service is being provide is no longer present, report the appropriate _______________ code as the first-listed or principal diagnosis.

18. For rehabilitation services following active treatment of an injury, assign the _________________ code with the appropriate seventh character for subsequent encounter as the first-listed or principal diagnosis.

19. For reporting purposes, the definition for "other diagnoses" is interpreted as additional conditions that affect patient care in terms of requiring:

    a. ____

    b. ____

    c. ____

    d. ____

    e. ____

20. The UHDDS item _________ defines Other Diagnoses as "all conditions that coexist at the time of admission, that develop subsequently, or that affect the treatment received and/or the length of stay.

21. Diagnoses that relate to an earlier episode which have no bearing on the current hospital stay are to be excluded.

    a. True
    b. False

22.   If a provider has included a previous diagnosis in the final diagnostic statement, such as the discharge summary or face sheet, it should ordinarily be coded.

a.   True
b.   False

23.   Some providers include in the diagnostic statement resolved conditions or diagnoses and status-post procedures from previous admissions that have no bearing on the current stay; such conditions are not to be reported and are coded only if required by ____

24.   When should history codes (categories Z80-Z87) be used as additional diagnoses?

____

____

____

25.   Abnormal findings are not coded and reported unless the provider indicates their clinical significance.

a.   True
b.   False

26.   If the findings are outside the normal range and the attending provider has ordered other tests to evaluate the condition or prescribed treatment, it is not appropriate to ask the provider whether the abnormal finding should be added.

a.   True
b.   False

27.   If the diagnosis documented at the time of discharge is qualified as "probable," "suspected," "likely," "questionable," "possible," or "still to be ruled out," "compatible with," "consistent with," or other similar terms indicating uncertainty, ______________ the condition as if it existed or was established.

Chapter 4-Outpatient Coding Guidelines

1. Outpatient coding guidelines have been approved for use by whom?

2. Guidelines in Section __________, Conventions, general coding guidelines and chapter-specific guidelines, should also be applied for outpatient services and office visits.

3. Information about the use of certain abbreviations, punctuation, symbols, and other conventions used in the ICD-10-CM Tabular list, can be found in Section ______ of these guidelines, under "Conventions Used in the Tabular List"

4. Section ______ contains general guidelines that apply to the entire classification.

5. Section ______ contains chapter specific guidelines that correspond to the chapters as they are arranged in the classification.

6. Information about the correct sequence to use in finding a code is also described in section ______.

7. The terms encounter and visit are often used interchangeably in describing outpatient service contacts, and therefore, appear together in the guidelines, without distinguishing one from the other.

   a. True
   b. False

8. The Uniform Hospital Discharge Data Set (UHDDS) definition of principal diagnosis applies to hospital-based outpatient services and provider-based office visits.

   a. True
   b. False

9.   Coding guidelines for inconclusive diagnoses (probable, suspected, rule out, etc.,) were developed for both inpatient and outpatient coding and reporting.

   a.   True
   b.   False

10.   In the outpatient setting, the term first-listed diagnosis is used in lieu of the:

   ____

11.   In determining the first-listed diagnosis, coding _______________ of ICD-10-CM, as well as the general and disease specific _____________ take precedence over the _____________ guidelines.

12.   Diagnoses often are not established at the time of the initial encounter/visit, it may take ____

   ____

13.   The most critical rule involves beginning the search for the correct code assignment through the ________________ Index; never begin searching initially in the _______________ list as this will lead to coding errors.

14.   When the patient presents for outpatient surgery, code the _________________ for the surgery as the first-listed diagnosis, even if the surgery is not performed due to a _______________________________.

15.   When a patient is admitted for observation for a medical condition, assign a code for the _______________________________ as the first-listed diagnosis.

16.   When a patient presents for outpatient surgery and develops complications requiring admission to observation, what is the first reported and secondary diagnosis?

   a.   ____

   b.   ____

17. Which codes must be used to identify diagnosis, symptoms, conditions, problems, complaints, or other reason(s) for the encounter/visit?

____

18. For accurate reporting of ICD-10-CM diagnosis codes, the documentation should describe the:

____

____

____

19. Codes that describe symptoms and signs, as opposed to diagnosis are acceptable when:

____

____

20. Which codes are used to deal with encounters for circumstances other than a disease or injury?

____

____

____

21. ICD-10-CM is composed of codes with_____, ______, ______, ______ and ______ characters.

22. A code is ____________________________ if it has not been coded to the full number of digits required for that code, including the 7th character, if applicable.

23. List first the ______________________________ code for the diagnosis, condition, problem, or other reason for the encounter shown in the medical record to be chiefly responsible for the services provided.

24.   What should be coded when a diagnosis is described as "probable" or "questionable" as an outpatient?

____

____

____

25.   ______________ diseases treated on an ongoing basis may be coded and reported as many times as the patient receives treatment and ________ for the condition(s).

26.   Code all documented conditions that coexist at the time of the encounter/visit, and require or affect patient care treatment or management.

   a.   True
   b.   False

27.   History codes (categories Z80-Z87) may not be used as secondary codes if the historical or family condition has an impact on current care or influences treatment.

   a.   True
   b.   False

28.   When a patient is receiving only diagnostic services during an encounter or visit, what should be the first listed diagnosis and what may be sequenced as additional diagnoses?

   a.   ____

         ____

         ____

   b.   ____

         ____

         ____

29.   For encounters for routine laboratory/radiology testing in the absence of any signs, symptoms, or the associated diagnosis, assign _________________.

30.   If routine testing is performed during the same encounter as a test to evaluate a sign, symptom, or diagnosis, it is appropriate to assign both the:

a.   ____

b.   ____

____

31.   For outpatient encounters for diagnostic tests that have been interpreted by a physician and the final report is available at the time of coding:

a.   What is coded?   ____

b.   What is not coded?   ____

32.   When a patient is receiving only therapeutic services during an encounter or visit, what should be the first listed diagnosis and what is sequenced as additional diagnoses?

a.   ____

____

____

____

____

____

b.   ____

33. The only exception is when the primary reason for the admission/encounter is chemotherapy, radiation therapy, the appropriate Z code for the service is listed first, and the diagnosis or problem for which the service is being performed second

    a. True
    b. False

34. When a patient is receiving preoperative evaluations only, what should be the first-listed diagnosis and what may be reported as an additional diagnosis or diagnoses?

    a. ____

    b. ____

       ____

    c. ____

       ____

35. For ambulatory surgery, code the diagnosis for which the surgery was performed.

    a. True
    b. False

36. If the postoperative diagnosis is known to be different from the preoperative diagnosis at the time the diagnosis is confirmed, select the ________________ diagnosis for coding, since it is most definitive.

37. The subcategories for encounters for general medical examinations, Z00.0- and encounter for routine child health examination, Z00.12-, provide codes for with and without ________________ findings.

38. Should a general medical examination result in an abnormal finding, the code for general medical examination with abnormal finding should be assigned as the ________________ diagnosis.

39.   An examination with abnormal findings refers to a condition/diagnosis that is newly identified or a change in severity of a chronic condition (such as uncontrolled hypertension, or an acute exacerbation of chronic obstructive pulmonary disease) during a routine physical examination.

a.   True
b.   False

Answer Key

Every effort has been made to ensure the accuracy of the answers below, please report all errors to
info@drlisalcampbell.org

Thank you!

Dr. Lisa L Campbell, PhD

Chapter 1-Conventions and General Coding Guidelines

Question	Answer
1	a. True
2	a. AHIMA b. AHA c. NCHS d. CMS
3	b. False
4	Coding; sequencing
5	Health Insurance Portability and Accountability Act (HIPAA)
6	Provider; coder
7	Record
8	Including hospital admissions
9	Diagnosis
10	(a) 1. Conventions for the ICD-10-CM, 2. General coding guidelines and 3. Chapter specific guidelines, (b) Selection of principal diagnosis, (c) Reporting additional diagnoses, (d) Diagnostic coding and reporting guidelines for outpatient services
11	b. False
12	all
13	Independent
14	Alphabetic Index, an alphabetical list of terms and their corresponding code, and the Tabular List, a chronological list of codes divided into chapters based on body system or condition.
15	a. the Index of Diseases and Injury b. the Index of External Causes of Injury, c. the Table of Neoplasms d. Table of Drugs and Chemicals.
16	a. True
17	3, 4, 5, 6 or 7 characters
18	Invalid
19	The ICD-10-CM uses an indented format for ease in reference.
20	For reporting purposes only codes are permissible, not categories or subcategories, and any applicable 7th character is required.
21	The ICD-10-CM utilizes a placeholder character "X".
22	a. True
23	7th
24	X

25	This abbreviation in the Alphabetic Index represents "other specified". When a specific code is not available for a condition, the Alphabetic Index directs the coder to the "other specified" code in the Tabular List.
26	This abbreviation is the equivalent of unspecified.
27	This abbreviation in the Tabular List represents "other specified". When a specific code is not available for a condition the Tabular List includes an NEC entry under a code to identify the code as the "other specified" code.
28	This abbreviation is the equivalent of unspecified.
29	(a) Used in Tabular List to enclose synonyms, alternative wording or explanatory phrases. Alphabetic Index to identify manifestation codes, (b) Alphabetic Index and Tabular List to enclosed supplementary words that may or may not, (c) Used in the Tabular List after an incomplete term that needs one or more of the modifiers
30	Codes titled "other" or "other specified" are for use when the information in the medical record provides detail for which a specific code does not exist.
31	Codes titled "unspecified" are for use when the information in the medical record is insufficient to assign a more specific code
32	Includes note
33	a. True
34	Two; different
35	That the code excluded should never be used at the same time as the code above the note.
36	Two
37	Unrelated
38	Excluded; both
39	Acceptable
40	Manifestation
41	Use additional code; manifestation
42	Principal diagnosis
43	a. True
44	"and" or "or"
45	"due to"
46	b. False
47	a. True
48	a. True
49	a. True
50	Referenced
51	a. True
52	Entries
53	a. True

54	A "code also" note instructs that two codes may be required to fully describe a condition, but this note does not provide sequencing direction, sequencing depends on the circumstances of the encounter.
55	Default code
56	Main; unspecified
57	The default code should be assigned.
58	Statement
59	Has
60	a. Tue
61	To select a code in the classification that corresponds to a diagnosis or reason for visit documented in a medical record, first locate the term in the Alphabetic Index, and then verify the code in the Tabular List.
62	Read; guided
63	A code
64	Tabular List
65	Required
66	Tabular List
67	Diagnosis
68	a. True
69	a. True
70	Codes from A00.0 through T88.9, Z00-Z99.8, U00-U85
71	Diagnosis
72	18
73	a. True
74	a. True
75	a. True
76	Infectious disease code
77	b. False
78	The casual condition is unknown or not applicable
79	Sequela, Complication, and Obstetric
80	Code both and sequence the acute (subacute) code first
81	(a) two diagnoses, (b) diagnosis with an associated secondary process (manifestation) and (c) diagnosis with an associated complication
82	Combination codes are identified by referring to subterm entries in the Alphabetic Index and by reading the inclusion and exclusion notes in the Tabular List.
83	Involved
84	a. True
85	a. True
86	Sequela

87	b. False
88	(a) The condition or nature of the late effect is sequenced first (b) the late effect code is sequenced second.
89	A manifestation code identified in the Tabular list and the title, or sequela code has been expanded to include the manifestation (s)
90	a. True
91	(a) If it did occur, code as confirmed diagnosis, (b) If it did not occur, reference the Alphabetic Index to determine if the condition has a subentry term for "impending" or "threatened" and also reference main term entries for "Impending" and for "Threatened." (c) If the sub-terms are listed, assign the given code (d) If the sub-terms are not listed, code the existing underlying condition(s) and not the condition described as impending or threatened
92	a. True
93	(a) Left, (b) Right, or (c) Bilateral
94	a. True
95	Unspecified
96	Bilateral
97	Unilateral
98	a. True
99	a. True
100	a. True
101	a. True
102	a. True
103	a. True
104	Clinicians; provider
105	a. True
106	b. False
107	Alphabetic index guidance
108	Integral
109	Relationship
110	a. True
111	a. True
112	a. False
113	a. True
114	uncertain
115	acceptable
116	a. True
117	Unspecified
118	a. True
119	b. False

120	External
121	Supplemental
122	Never
123	a. How the injury or health condition happened (cause) b. Intent (unintentional or accidental; or intentional, such as suicide or assault) c. Place where the event occurred d. Activity of the patient at the time of the event e. Person's status (e.g., civilian, military)
124	b. False
125	a. True
126	a. True
127	a. True
128	Cataclysmic
129	Many
130	Hurricane
131	Levee
132	Flooding
133	a. True
134	a. True
135	a. True
136	Hurricane
137	Explain

Chapter 2-Chapter Specific Coding Guidelines

C1-Certain Infectious and Parasitic Disease-(A00-B99, U07.1)

Question	Answer
1	You should only code confirmed cases of HIV infection/illness
2	b. False
3	a. Principal diagnosis should be B20 b. Additional diagnosis codes for all reported HIV related condition
4	D59.31
5	a. Code for the unrelated condition should be the principal diagnosis b. B20, followed by additional diagnosis codes
6	b. False
7	a. HIV positive, b. Known HIV c. HIV test positive d. Similar terminology
8	a. True
9	Patients with inconclusive HIV serology but no definitive diagnosis or manifestations of the illness
10	B20
11	a. True
12	b. True
13	a. 098.7- b. B20
14	a. O98.7- b. Z21
15	Z11.4
16	Signs and symptoms
17	Z71.7
18	a. True
19	a. False
20	b. False
21	A41.9
22	Severe sepsis or an associated acute organ dysfunction is documented
23	a. True
24	Nonspecific term
25	Severe sepsis

26	a. False
27	The severe sepsis code
28	a. True
29	a. True
30	a. True
31	Represents a type of acute organ dysfunction
32	a. Code for the systemic infection b. R65.21 or T81.12
33	b. False
34	Subcategory R65.2, Secondary diagnoses
35	a. True
36	R65.2; secondary diagnosis
37	Confirmed
38	a. Underlying systemic infection b. Localized infection
39	a. localized infection b. sepsis/severe sepsis code
40	Infection; procedure
41	a. True
42	a. True
43	Infection
44	a. True
45	a. noninfectious condition b. Infection
46	Noninfectious
47	a. True
48	A code from subcategory R65.1, Systemic inflammatory response syndrome (SIRS) of non-infectious origin.
49	a. True
50	Code
51	B95.62
52	Colonization or carriage
53	a. True
54	a. True
55	Z22.322
56	Z22.321
57	a. True
58	a. True
59	Confirmed
60	a. True

61	a. True
62	Confirmed
63	a. True
64	a. True
65	a. True
66	U07.1
67	Additional
68	U07.1, J20.8
69	U07.1, J40
70	U07.1, J22
71	U07.1, J98.8
72	U07.1, J80
73	U07.1, J96.0-
74	a. True
75	Asymptomatic
76	Symptomatic
77	Each
78	b. False
79	b. False
80	Z09, Z86.16
81	Z01.84

C2-Neoplasms (C00-D49)

Question	Answer
1	(a) benign, (b) in-situ, (c) malignant, (d) uncertain histologic behavior
2	The combination is specifically indexed elsewhere.
3	a. True
4	Ectopic Tissues
5	b. False
6	Tabular list
7	malignancy
8	Z51. --
9	The secondary neoplasm is designated as the principal diagnosis even though the primary malignancy is still present
10	a. The appropriate malignancy code b. D63.0, Anemia in neoplastic disease
11	a. Anemia b. Neoplasm c. Adverse effect
12	Y84.2
13	a. Dehydration b. Malignancy
14	Designate the complication as the principal or first-listed diagnosis if treatment is directed at resolving the complication
15	a. True
16	Secondary
17	Neoplasm
18	a. Z51.0, Encounter for antineoplastic radiation therapy b. Z51.11, Encounter for antineoplastic chemotherapy c. Z51.12, Encounter for antineoplastic immunotherapy as the first listed or principal diagnosis
19	a. True
20	a. Z51.0, Encounter for antineoplastic radiation therapy b. Z51.11, Encounter for antineoplastic chemotherapy c. Z51.12, Encounter for antineoplastic immunotherapy as the first listed or principal diagnosis
21	Malignancy
22	Metastatic
23	b. False
24	b. False

25	a. True
26	a. True
27	Malignancy
28	The metastatic site(s)
29	a. True
30	b. False
31	D63.0, Anemia in Neoplastic Disease
32	Principal/first-listed diagnosis
33	M84.5, Pathological fracture in neoplastic disease, the code for the neoplasm
34	neoplasm code should be sequenced first, pathological fracture
35	a. True
36	A code from category Z85, Personal history of malignant neoplasm, should be used to indicate the former site of the malignancy
37	Secondary
38	Primary; Secondary
39	a. True
40	Transplanted, T86-, C80.2, malignancy
41	9

C4-Endocrine, Nutritional and Metabolic Disease (E00-E89)

Question	Answer
1	a. the type of diabetes mellitus b. the body system affected c. the complications affecting the body system
2	Reason
3	a. True
4	b. False
5	E11.-, Type 2 diabetes mellitus
6	a. True
7	Insulin
8	Z79.4, Z79.85
9	Z79.84, Z79.85
10	a. True
11	a. T85.6, Mechanical complication due to insulin pump b. T38.3x6-, Underdosing of insulin and oral hypoglycemic drugs
12	a. T85.6-, Mechanical complication of other specified internal and external prosthetic devices, implants and grafts b. T38.3x1-, Poisoning by insulin and oral hypoglycemic drugs, accidental
13	Secondary
14	b. False
15	Z79
16	Both
17	Tabular List instructions for categories E08, E09 and E13.
18	a. E89.1, Postprocedural hypoinsulinemia b. E13 c. Z90.41-, Acquired absence of pancreas, as additional codes
19	a. True

C5-Mental and Behavioral Disorders (F01-F99)

Question	Answer
1	a. True
2	Category G89, Pain, not elsewhere classified, if there is documentation of a psychological component for a patient with acute or chronic pain.
3	Clinical judgment
4	Remission
5	a. If both use and abuse are documented, assign only the code for abuse b. If both abuse and dependence are documented, assign only the code for dependence, c. If use, abuse, and dependence are all documented, assign only the code for dependence, d. If both use and dependence are documented, assign only the code for dependence.
6	a. True
7	b. False
8	a. True
9	b. False
10	a. True
11	a. True
12	a. True
13	F68.A
14	T74, T76
15	a. Unspecified b. mild c. moderate d. severe
16	Unspecified
17	b. False

C6-Diseases of Nervous System and Sense Organs (G00-G99)

Question	Answer
1	Identify whether the dominant or nondominant side is affected.
2	(a) For ambidextrous patients, the default should be dominant, (b) If the left side is affected, the default is non-dominant, (c) If the right side is affected, the default is dominant.
3	a. acute or chronic pain b. neoplasm related pain
4	G89
5	Underlying condition
6	Principal
7	a. When pain control or pain management is the reason for the admission/encounter (e.g., a patient with displaced intervertebral disc, nerve impingement and severe back pain presents for injection of steroid into the spinal canal). The underlying cause of the pain should be reported as an additional diagnosis, if known b. When a patient is admitted for the insertion of a neurostimulator for pain control, assign the appropriate pain code as the principal or first listed diagnosis. When an admission or encounter is for a procedure aimed at treating the underlying condition and a neurostimulator is inserted for pain control during the same admission/encounter, a code for the underlying condition should be assigned as the principal diagnosis and the appropriate pain code should be assigned as a secondary diagnosis
8	Information
9	a. Code from category G89 b. Code identifying the specific site of pain
10	The appropriate code from category G89
11	Provider's
12	Acute form
13	b. False
14	Category G89
15	The appropriate code(s) found in Chapter 19, Injury, poisoning and certain other consequences of external causes
16	G89.2
17	G89.3
18	Control/management
19	a. True
20	a. True

C7-Diseases of the Eye and Adnexa (H00-H59)

Question	Answer
1	(a) type of glaucoma, (b) the affected eye, (c) and the glaucoma stage.
2	Report only the code for the type of glaucoma, bilateral, with the seventh character for the stage.
3	Report only one code for the type of glaucoma with the appropriate seventh character for the stage.
4	a. True
5	Seventh
6	a. True
7	b. False
8	Clinical documentation
9	Clinically
10	0
11	a. True
12	a. True
13	a. True

C9-Disease of the Circulatory System (I00-I99)

Question	Answer
1	a. True
2	a. True
3	a. True
4	Hypertension
5	I50
6	a. True
7	Are present
8	CKD
9	N18
10	Hypertensive chronic kidney disease
11	Hypertension, heart; kidney
12	a. True
13	Combination
14	I13
15	Coded
16	a. First assign codes from I60-I69 b. Followed by the appropriate hypertension code
17	Sequencing
18	a. one to identify the underlying etiology b. one from category I15 to identify the hypertension
19	Hypertension
20	a. True
21	Control
22	Responding
23	Urgency, emergency, reason
24	Sequencing
25	a. I25.11 b. I25.7
26	a. True
27	Atherosclerosis; angina pectoris
28	Coronary artery disease
29	b. False
30	Type
31	I60-I67
32	Onset

33	Arise; onset
34	Dominant; nondominant
35	a. for ambidextrous patients, the default should be dominant b. If the left side is affected, the default is non-dominant c. If the right side is affected, the default is dominant
36	Deficits
37	a. True
38	a. True
39	I21.3
40	I21.4
41	STEMI
42	a. True
43	a. True
44	a. True
45	I25.2
46	a. True
47	Type 1
48	Subendocardial AMI
49	Four
50	a. True
51	b. False
52	I22
53	I21.A1
54	I21.A9
55	I21
56	I22
57	1
58	2
59	Demand
60	Circumstances
61	I21.A1
62	a. True
63	a. True
64	b. False

C10-Diseases of Respiratory System (J00-J99)

Question	Answer
1	J44 and J45
2	a. True
3	It is the condition established after study to be chiefly responsible for occasioning the admission to the hospital and the selection is supported by the Alphabetic Index and Tabular List
4	Secondary diagnosis
5	Will not be the same in every situation
6	Terms found in Alphabetical Index
7	Query the provider for clarification
8	a. True
9	b. False
10	Category J11 should be assigned
11	Condition; procedure
12	a. True
13	a. True
14	a. True
15	a. True
16	Categories J12-J18 for the pneumonia diagnosed at the time of admission
17	a. True
18	Principal
19	U07.0
20	a. True

C12-Diseases of Skin and Subcutaneous Tissue (L00-L99)

Question	Answer
1	Stage
2	a. Stage 1-4 b. unspecified stage c. unstageable
3	Identify
4	a. True
5	Unspecified stage, (L89.- -9)
6	Pressure ulcer stage codes are based on the documentation in the medical record
7	a. True
8	Healing
9	The appropriate code for unspecified stage
10	a. True
11	Present
12	a. one code for the site and stage of the ulcer on admission b. second code for the same ulcer site and the highest stage reported during the hospital stay
13	a. True
14	Healed
15	Healing
16	Severity
17	Query
18	a. True
19	a. one code for the site b. severity level of the ulcer on admission and a second code for the same ulcer and the highest severity level reported during the stay

C13-Diseases of Musculoskeletal and Connective Tissue (M00-M99)

Question	Answer
1	b. False
2	The site represents the bone, joint or the muscle involved.
3	a. True
4	Chapter 13; Chapter 19
5	a. True
6	a. True
7	The appropriate complication codes
8	Of the codes under category M81
9	Pathologic
10	Z87.310
11	Pathologic
12	Site
13	M80

C14-Diseases of Genitourinary System (N00-N99)

Question	Answer
1	1-5
2	Mild CKD
3	Moderate CKD
4	Severe CKD
5	N18.6
6	Code N18.6 only
7	The kidney transplant may not fully restore kidney function
8	Z94.0
9	Query the provider
10	Tabular List

C15- Pregnancy, Childbirth and the Puerperium (O00-O9A)

Question	Answer
1	b. False
2	Z33.1
3	b. False
4	Trimester of the pregnancy
5	a. True
6	b. False
7	Antepartum complication
8	The trimester character for the trimester at the time of the admission/encounter should be assigned.
9	a. True
10	(a) For single gestations, (b) When the documentation in the record is insufficient to determine the fetus affected and it is not possible to obtain clarification, (c) When it is not possible to clinically determine which fetus is affected.
11	Completed
12	A code from category Z34
13	a. True
14	Labor; delivery
15	O80
16	High Risk
17	First
18	Sequenced
19	Additional
20	Cesarean
21	Unrelated
22	record
23	a. True
24	a. True
25	Secondary
26	a. True
27	b. False
28	Fetal
29	a. True
30	O98.7-, HIV-related
31	O98.7- and Z21

32	a. Category O24, Diabetes mellitus in pregnancy, childbirth and the puerperium first b. followed by the appropriate diabetes codes(s) (E08-E13) from Chapter 4
33	a. True
34	a. diet controlled b. insulin controlled c. controlled by oral hypoglycemic drugs
35	a. True
36	b. False
37	Specific type of infection
38	Should be assigned as an additional diagnosis
39	The casual organism
40	a. True
41	F10
42	F17
43	F11-F16 and F18-F19
44	a. True
45	a. full-term normal delivery b. single, healthy infant c. without any complications antepartum complication, during the delivery, or postpartum during the delivery episode
46	a. True
47	Had a complication at some point during her pregnancy but the complication is not present at the time of the admission for delivery
48	Z37.0, Single live birth
49	Immediately after delivery and continues for six weeks following delivery
50	Month; five
51	Is any complication occurring within the six week period
52	a. True
53	Z39.0
54	a. True
55	The cardiomyopathy develops as a result of pregnancy in a women who did not have pre-existing heart disease
56	Initial complication of a pregnancy develops a sequelae requiring care or treatment at a future date
57	Anytime after the initial postpartum period
58	This code like all late effect codes is to be sequenced following the code describing the sequel of the complication
59	a. Z33.2 b. Z37.0

60	a. Category O03.4, Spontaneous abortion b. O07.4, Failed attempted termination of pregnancy without complications c. Z33.2, Encounter for elective termination of pregnancy
61	a. True
62	O04, O07 and O08
63	O04.6
64	b. False
65	O98.5-
66	O98.5- and U07.1

Newborn (Perinatal) Guidelines (P00-P96)

Question	Answer
1	Birth; 28th
2	b. False
3	a. True
4	b. False
5	Once
6	a. True
7	a. True
8	Detail
9	a. True
10	a. True
11	Due to the birth process and the code from chapter 16 should be used
12	(a) Clinical evaluation (b) therapeutic treatment, (c) diagnostic procedure, (d) extended length of hospital stay, (e) increasing nursing care and/or monitoring, (f) has implication for future health care needs
13	a. True
14	Z05
15	a. True
16	Z38
17	a. True
18	Secondary
19	b. False
20	a. True
21	It is documented
22	Weigh; gestational
23	Birth weight
24	a. True
25	P36
26	B95
27	a. True
28	a. True
29	a. True
30	b. False

C17-Congenital Malformations, Deformations, and Chromosomal Abnormalities (Q00-Q99)

Question	Answer
1	Chromosomal abnormality
2	a. True
3	Unique
4	Inherent
5	b. False
6	b. False
7	Later in life
8	a. True
9	Principal

C18-Symptoms, Signs, Abnormal Clinical & Lab Findings, (R00-R99)

Question	Answer
1	Diagnosis
2	a. True
3	May
4	a. True
5	Definitive; common
6	R29.6
7	Z91.81
8	a. True
9	a. True
10	Sequenced
11	a. True
12	a. True
13	R65.10; R65.11
14	acute organ dysfunction
15	Queried
16	b. False
17	Conjunction
18	After

C19-Injury, Poisoning, and Other Consequences of External Causes (S00-T88)

Question	Answer
1	7th
2	a. True
3	Additional
4	Active; seeing
5	a. True
6	A
7	D
8	a. True
9	S
10	Injury; sequela
11	Sequela; injury
12	a. True
13	Inpatient
14	b. False
15	a. True
16	Not coded
17	b. False
18	Primary
19	a. True
20	Individually
21	Open; Closed
22	Displaced; not displaced
23	Traumatic
24	Initial
25	a. True
26	a. True
27	a. True
28	7th character
29	Gustilo
30	a. True
31	a. True
32	7th character
33	Severity of the fracture
34	a. True
35	Burn
36	Chemicals

37	b. False
38	Depth, Extent, Agent
39	First degree, second degree, and third degree
40	Site
41	First
42	Sequence first
43	Admission
44	b. False
45	Highest
46	Acute
47	a. True
48	Additional
49	Separate
50	Extremely, rarely
51	a. True
52	Burn mortality
53	Third-degree
54	"Rule of Nines" in estimating body surface involved
55	With a burn or corrosion code with the 7th character "S" for sequela
56	"A" or "D"
57	External cause
58	Combination
59	b. False
60	b. False
61	a. True
62	b. False
63	Combination code
64	a. assign the appropriate code for the nature of the adverse effect b. code for the adverse effect of the drug (T36-T50)
65	T36-T50
66	Accidental
67	a. True
68	Additional code
69	Principal
70	Relapse
71	a. True
72	Toxic
73	a. accidental b. intentional self-harm

	c. assault
	d. undetermined
74	a. True
75	T74.-; T76-
76	X92-Y09
77	A perpetrator code
78	a. True
79	a. True
80	Z04.81; Z04.82
81	Pain
82	T codes; G89
83	Complications
84	The function of the transplanted organ
85	a. The appropriate code from category T86
	b. Secondary code that identifies the complication
86	Affect the function of the transplanted organs
87	T86.1-
88	kidney
89	Query the provider
90	a. T86.1
	b. Secondary code that identifies the complication
91	a. True
92	a. True
93	a. True

C20-External Causes of Morbidity (V01-Y99)

Question	Answer
1	a. True
2	b. False
3	a. how the injury or health condition happened (cause), b. the intent (unintentional or accidental; or intentional, such as suicide or assault), c. the place where the event occurred d. the activity of the patient at the time of the event, and e. the person's status (e.g., civilian, military)
4	An external cause code may be used with any code in the range of A00.0-T88.9, Z00-Z99, classification that is a health condition due to an external cause.
5	b. False, with the 7th character
6	7th; A; D; S
7	Match
8	Full
9	Explain each cause
10	To the principal diagnosis
11	Alphabetic index
12	a. True
13	b. False, they should correspond to the sequence of events.
14	b. False, they should not be used if included in another chapter.
15	The location of the patient at the time of injury or other condition.
16	a. True
17	b. False, no 7th characters are used
18	b. False
19	Y93
20	a. True
21	a. True
22	b. False
23	a. True
24	Y93
25	The main external cause codes
26	a. place of occurrence code; b. one activity code; and c. one external cause status code assigned to an encounter
27	Principal diagnosis
28	Cause/intent

29	(a) child and abuse (b) terrorism events , (c) cataclysmic events, (d) transport accidents, (e) activity, (f) first-listed
30	Assault
31	From Y07, Perpetrator of maltreatment
32	Accidental intent
33	transport
34	a. True
35	S; should
36	Current
37	Treated
38	Injury
39	Y38
40	Is found at the inclusion note at the beginning of category Y38
41	a. True
42	Y38
43	Assault
44	Assign code Y38.9
45	a. False, it is acceptable
46	Should
47	Work status
48	a. military activity; b. whether a non-military person was at work; c. whether an individual including a student or volunteer was involved in a non-work activity at the time of the causal event.
49	a. True
50	a. poisonings; b. adverse effects; c. misadventures or d. late effects.
51	If no other external cause codes
52	Once
53	a. True
54	a. True

C21-Factors Influencing Health Status and Contact with Health Services (Z00-Z99)

Question	Answer
1	a. True
2	Certain
3	b. False
4	Corresponding
5	Z20
6	Suspected
7	Z77
8	First-listed
9	Inoculations; vaccinations
10	Procedure
11	Secondary
12	Status
13	Treatment and its outcome
14	No
15	b. False
16	Weaning
17	a. True
18	Susceptible
19	a. follow-up code should be sequenced first, b. followed by the appropriate personal history and genetic susceptibility codes.
20	Z15
21	Z16
22	Z21
23	Z22
24	Secondary
25	Z66
26	Reportable
27	a. True
28	Continuous; medication
29	Z92.82
30	a. True
31	Personal; family
32	Personal
33	Family

34	Personal; family
35	a. True
36	Present
37	Screening
38	Diagnostic examination
39	First; screening
40	Inherent
41	Condition
42	Planned; performed
43	Very
44	Injury; illness
45	a. True
46	Unrelated
47	a. True
48	First listed; ruled
49	a. True
50	b. False
51	Initial
52	a. True
53	7th
54	First listed
55	Reason; diagnosis
56	Directed
57	Condition or sequelae
58	Z
59	Status
60	Fully; exists
61	Aftercare
62	a. True
63	Diagnosis
64	a. True
65	Counseling
66	a. True
67	Not
68	Additional; pregnancy
69	a. True
70	Date
71	a. True
72	Z37

73	Family planning
74	a. True
75	a. True
76	Administrative
77	Time
78	Identify
79	a. True
80	a. Code from category Z40, Encounter for prophylactic surgery, b. Appropriate codes to identify the associated risk factor
81	a. True
82	Z40.0
83	Inpatient; Outpatient; more precise coding
84	Documented
85	Many

Chapter 3-Selection of Principal and Secondary Diagnoses

Question	Answer
1	The condition established after study to be chiefly responsible for occasioning the admission of the patient to the hospital for care.
2	b. False
3	a. True
4	Application; impossible
5	a. True
6	Either condition may be sequenced first, unless the circumstances of the admission the therapy provided, the Tabular List or Alphabetic Index indicate otherwise.
7	Diagnoses
8	They are coded as if the diagnoses were confirmed and the diagnoses are sequenced according to the circumstance of the admission
9	Sequence as the principal diagnosis the condition which after study occasioned the admission to the hospital, even though treatment may not have been carried out due to unforeseen circumstances
10	The complication code
11	a. True
12	Code the condition as if it existed or was established
13	The medical condition which led to the hospital admission
14	Principal diagnosis
15	(a) If the reason for the inpatient admission is a complication, assign the complication as the principal diagnosis. (b) If no complication or other condition is documented as the reason for the inpatient admission, assign the reason for the outpatient surgery as the principal diagnosis. (c) If the reason for the inpatient admission is another condition unrelated to the surgery, assign the unrelated condition as the principal diagnosis.
16	a. True
17	aftercare
18	Injury
19	(a) clinical evaluation, (b) therapeutic treatment, (c) diagnostic procedures, (d) extended length of stay, (e) increased nursing care and/or monitoring
20	11-b
21	a. True
22	a. True
23	Hospital policy
24	If the historical condition or family history has an impact on current care or influences treatment
25	a. True

26	b. False
27	Code

Chapter 4-Outpatient Coding and Reporting

Question	Answer
1	These coding guidelines for outpatient diagnoses have been approved for use by hospitals/ providers in coding and reporting hospital-based outpatient services and provider-based office visits.
2	Section I
3	Section IA
4	Section IB
5	Section IC
6	Section I
7	a. True
8	b. False
9	b. False
10	Principal
11	Conventions; guidelines; outpatient
12	Two or more visits before the diagnosis is confirmed
13	Alphabetical; Tabular
14	Reason; contraindication
15	Medical condition
16	Reason for the surgery; complications
17	A00.0 through T88.9, Z00-Z99, U00-U85
18	The patient's condition using terminology which includes specific diagnoses as well as symptoms, problems or reason for the encounter
19	Codes that describe symptoms and signs, as opposed to diagnoses, are acceptable for reporting purposes when a diagnosis has not been established (confirmed) by the provider.
20	The Factors Influencing Health Status and Contact with Health Services codes (Z00-Z99) are provided to deal with occasions when occasions when circumstances other than a disease or injury are recorded as diagnosis or problems.
21	3, 4, 5, 6 or 7
22	Invalid
23	ICD-10-CM
24	Code the condition(s) to the highest degree of certainty for that encounter/visit, such as symptoms, signs, abnormal test results, or other reason for the visit.
25	Chronic, care

26	a. True
27	b. False
28	a. Condition, problem, or other reason for encounter/or visit shown in medical record, b. codes for other diagnoses may be sequenced as additional diagnosis
29	Z01.89, Encounter for other specified special examinations
30	a. Z code and b. the code describing the reason for the non-routine test
31	a. Code any confirmed or definitive diagnosis (es) documented in the interpretation; b. do not code related signs and symptoms as additional diagnoses.
32	a. Sequence first the diagnosis condition, problem or other reason for encounter/visit shown in the medical record. b. Codes for other diagnoses may be sequenced as additional diagnoses
33	a. True
34	a. First a code from subcategory Z01.81 for the pre-op consultation. b. Assign a code for the condition to describe the reason for the surgery as an additional diagnosis c. Code also any findings related to the pre-op evaluation
35	a. True
36	Postoperative
37	Abnormal
38	First listed
39	a. True